OPENING BOXES

How to Navigate Life When You Have Autism

Jay Rothman

Improving Your Life Publishing House
2025

Copyright ©2025 Jay Rothman
Improving Your Life Publishing House

All rights reserved. No part of this publication may be used without the prior written permission of the publisher.

Cover Designer: Laura Orsini
Front Cover Artist: Elena Tarsius
Back Cover Photographer: Jennifer Rebhan

Rothman, Jay, 1961 – author.

Opening Boxes: How to Navigate Life When You Have Autism / Jay Rothman.

ISBN 979-8-9921654-0-1

First Edition

Printed in the United States of America

Contents

Dedications v

Acknowledgments vii

Preface ix

Opening 1

1. Reality Is What I Say It Is 3
2. Why Are Relationships So Difficult to Build? 9
3. Dreams and Aspirations 19
4. Positivity Despite Life-Altering Diseases 23
5. Surrounded by Bullies 27
6. Employment 33
7. Personal Employment Challenges 41
8. Managing Your Money 45
9. "Disconnection" and the Increasing Number of People on the Spectrum 53
10. Subtext/Be Smart/We Are Not Robots 57
11. How to Develop Friendships 61
12. The Positive Side 65
13. Sugarcoated 69
14. Faulty Connections 71
15. Eliminate Sadness 75

16. Live a Balanced Life 81
17. Autism and Sensitivity 83
18. Autism and OCD 87
19. Stuck in the Past 91
20. Autism and Depression 93
21. It's Time to See a Therapist 97
22. It's OK to Be Different (Follow Your Own Path) 101
23. Don't Be a Sucker 103
24. Be Wise 107
25. Happiness 109
26. Concluding Thoughts 111
Endnotes.. 113

Dedications

Nathan Stanley Kolker: Reach for the basket, drive toward your dreams.

Joanna Elizabeth Kolker: Can you hear me?

Paul Kirkman: "Put a little magic in your life."

Heather Olsen: Healing Angel.

Acknowledgments

I offer thanks to Marlene Maschan, my mother; Larry Rothman, my deceased father; and Jerry Maschan, my deceased stepfather, for their roles in molding me into the person I am. My parents wanted the best for me, although many times my autism got in the way of my success. I also thank Paul Kirkman, whom I met in my freshman year at the University of Missouri-Columbia. He taught me magic tricks and philosophy, and even though we practice different religions, lit my path, enabling me to become much more interested in learning about my own faith.

In addition, Heather Olsen, an energy healer with psychic and medium abilities, who lives in Pennsylvania, has done wonders for my self-esteem and self-worth. I credit her for helping me break through my negativity and showing me a better life path. Now I can see much more positive potential than downfalls in my future. She is an inspiration. Heather can be reached at **TruHealingCenter.com**.

Applause is also extended to Susan Golubock, Dr. Temple Grandin, Paul Kirkman, Nathan Kolker, and Heather Olsen for sharing their thoughts about my book before publication.

I also thank Dr. Grandin for including my chapter in her book, *Different...Not Less*, 2nd edition.

Preface

Thank you for choosing to read this book. There are many options to deepen your awareness of autism. I am honored you are allowing me into your world.

In 2008, at the age of 46, I was diagnosed with autism. Most people might have been pleased to learn there was a logical reason for why the world responded to them as it did. I was not happy because I was stuck with another label, another wall that separated me from everyone else. In reality, that wall had always been there, be it named or not. I was always different from my peers, never feeling I fit in. By receiving a diagnosis, I learned who I am and was, then able to learn how to break through each communication barrier, one at a time. Once I shattered the impasses that blocked my every step, I wanted to share my experiences, in the hope that this information might help guide others to overcome obstacles with less difficulty.

My intention is to bring those with autism and those not on the autism spectrum closer together. There are definite differences in how both groups think and relate to the world. These differences, when understood, are not insurmountable. My goal is to provide a roadmap to improve communication between both groups, exploring ways for those on the autism spectrum to move more smoothly through life. This book will also teach neurotypicals (a term for those not on the autism spectrum) how we think, as well as parents and educators, so they can help guide us.

In terms of communication, both sides need to move as close to the center as they are able. Sometimes, a person on the spectrum can be flexible; other times, little movement will occur. It is important for each individual to try to understand the other person's feelings and not expect the other person to do all the work. Growth can occur when you leave your comfort zone. Take a chance and move forward. If the forward movement is too far, step back a little and contemplate why you are uncomfortable. Maybe you will be able to move forward, maybe not.

There are several things a person with autism can do to improve communication:

1. Tell neurotypicals what you need from them. This is called advocating for yourself.
2. Expand your perspective and talk about the other person's interests.
3. Compromise, taking your friend's/partner's needs into consideration.
4. Work on having a small amount of eye contact with the person you are speaking to.
5. Go as far as you are able. I write in more detail about these topics in the following chapters.

What can a non-autistic person do to improve communication with someone on the spectrum?

1. Tell us what is important to you but realize we may not have the ability to do what you want. For example, those on the autism spectrum can rarely look at you and speak to you at the same time. Even though it is very easy for a non-autistic to do, this is very difficult for someone on the spectrum.
2. Understand that being patient with autistics will improve communication with us and help keep us from closing up.
3. Be literal. Say exactly what you mean and avoid using subtext with a person on the spectrum. Subtext is the unspoken real meaning of words. We often don't understand subtext because autistics only understand the words that are spoken.
4. Remember that autistics cannot comprehend or express body language. Personally, I am told that my face is "expressionless."
5. Give us time to process questions. Avoid demanding immediate answers.
6. Recognize that autistics have a better understanding of what you are communicating when it is visual, not verbal.

One area with a high rate of failure between those on the autism spectrum and neurotypicals is long-term relationships. The divorce rate for people with autism is approximately 80 percent.[1] In *Chapter 2: Why Are Relationships So Difficult to Build?*, I offer advice to both groups about how to work with their partner to create a clear understanding of each person's wants and needs. Communication, flexibility, and seeing the world from the other person's point of view are very important for those both on and off the spectrum.

I also share my thoughts about how to avoid life's obstacles for those on the spectrum. In *Chapter 6: Employment*, a few of the topics I cover are getting along with others, teamwork, listening, and doing your best. Understanding proper social interactions can help people with autism avoid problems in the workplace and in all areas of life. *Chapter 11: How to Develop Friendships* reminds readers what a good friend does for another friend. In *Chapter 23: Don't Be a Sucker*, I share some of the bad situations I almost fell into.

Some of these thoughts might appear to be basic knowledge for a person not on the autism spectrum. After all, they picked up this information when they were very young. Who doesn't know this stuff? Autistic people don't, which is why we have so many difficulties in life.

Being on the spectrum is not rare or unusual. An estimated 5,437,988 adults 18 years of age or older, or 2.21 percent of the United States population, has autism spectrum disorder, according to a 2017 study published in May 2020 by the Centers for Disease Control and Prevention (CDC).[2] Because it is becoming more common for those on the spectrum and neurotypicals to interact with each other, both groups must learn how to better communicate with each other.

This book is different from other books about autism because it explains how to move through life more smoothly in four ways.

First, rather than stopping at the basics of employment, money and relationships, I extend my advice to often-ignored areas, such as sharing your gifts with the world rather than staying closed up.

Second, I also provide instruction about how to fulfill your dreams or goals in life. *Chapter 3: Dreams and Aspirations* provides guidance on how to transform your life into what you want it to be.

Third, I share short stories about my life, rather than writing an entire chapter about a single event, like several other books about autism do. I find it important to relay my ideas in a few paragraphs that get straight to the point.

Fourth, many people look at the dark side of life, rather than seeing the positive aspects. I encourage you to open your heart to gratitude, because doing so will dissolve the clouds so you will feel warm rays of light in your physical world and in your heart. Happiness brings forth joy, while sadness brings a dreariness to your life and your soul.

My father used to say, "You can always look up and you can always look down." He meant that others are both better off and worse off than you. Be grateful for what you have.

I titled this book *Opening Boxes: How to Navigate Life When You Have Autism* because I was stuck living in my own world, a closed-off world, for many decades. It was a world I could neither have anyone enter, nor could I leave. I was, for all essential purposes, in a closed box.

Now that I am older and have had years of therapy, I have the ability to open the box and interact with the world, no longer feeling the need to hide to keep myself safe from others. I am now able to allow my readers and brand-new acquaintances into my world.

I am much more than a person with autism. Just like everyone else on the spectrum, I have dreams and goals. My opportunities are endless. I have been through heavy downpours and can finally see a rainbow of hope in front of me.

Life can be quite challenging for those on the autism spectrum. With much work, we can overcome our obstacles.

Opening

Living in a box alone is difficult when you realize there is a world outside your box that you want to be a part of.

Chapter 1

Reality Is What I Say It Is

It was 2008 when I became aware that I have a condition called autism spectrum disorder (at the time, it was called Asperger's syndrome). For the previous 46 years, I knew I was different – very different – from my family, the few friends I had, and everyone else. I just didn't know this difference had a name or that I wasn't the only person who was so different from everyone else.

Autism spectrum disorder means that its severity varies for people on the spectrum. Signs of ASD include lack of eye contact, intense interest in a single subject, inability to cope with changes in routine, and being unable to understand another person's feelings. Characteristic of everyone on the spectrum is a lack of social skills. That is one of the primary ways I am different: I feel out of place within the rest of society.

Not fitting in is not a problem until you become tired of being the outsider. The person no one understands. The one who has no friends. The one in a box.

I was not accepted by others. My stepfather labeled me "eccentric." He was being kind. Most everyone I knew either ignored me or talked about me behind my back. Some were just cruel.

In 2008, while at my doctor's office, a phlebotomist was taking blood from my arm when I flinched because of the needle. She harshly said, "If you do that, I will get stuck."

I retorted, "Better you than me."

She described my behavior to my doctor as violent and told her I tried to harm her. I had not. No matter. I received a typed certified letter informing me that I was being dismissed from my doctor's practice. My psychiatrist tried to intervene, to no avail.

I felt embarrassed and misunderstood. The phlebotomist had been verbally abusive and unfriendly before I flinched, and yet I was the one blamed and ultimately penalized. She perceived me as threatening her. I believed she was being mean to me.

According to the *Diagnostic and Statistical Manual of Mental Disorders* (DSM-5), published by the American Psychiatric Association, "Older individuals may struggle to understand what behavior is considered appropriate in one situation but not another."[3]

* * *

Miscommunication is a constant in my life. Many people see me as rigid, unfriendly, and rude, while I find the world thoughtless of my feelings, insensitive, and difficult to understand.

Why are our perspectives so different? Those with autism have weaker social skills than neurotypicals. Without the ability to interpret the subtleties of spoken language and body language, we are lost. I liken it to trying to use a map without understanding what the symbols mean. Would you be able to find your way to your destination? Probably not.

Both spoken language and body language are languages unto themselves, and most communication is non-verbal. Autistics miss things like eye movements, inflection in a person's voice, positioning of arms and legs, and subtext (the true meaning of words). It seems like nearly everyone else is on the same page, while those on the autism spectrum are reading from a different book.

Attempting to fit in is all we can do because we are uncomfortable in the neurotypical world. The chitchat and not-saying-what-you-mean world of neurotypical communication is a mystery. Attempting to conform begets stress and unease.

Often, no matter how hard we try, we cannot merge completely into the neurotypical world. I liken it to the gauntlet braces I wear on both my legs and feet. If I tried to run a marathon, it would be a miracle for me to finish one-tenth of a mile; completing 26.2 miles would never be possible. Those of us with ASD can try our best to join the non-autistic world, as long as neurotypicals realize that we cannot fit in smoothly or for very long.

As mentioned above, miscommunication is constant. I was scheduled to stay in a hotel for an extended period because of damage to my home. Nine days after I checked in, they asked me to check out. They never explained the reason, but it probably had to do with miscommunication with the housekeeper and/or the general manager.

The maintenance man was already in my hotel room when the housekeeper walked in. I told her what I needed, and she said, "No English." This caught me off-guard. I asked the maintenance man if he could translate for me. He did, and so she vacuumed and emptied the trash. The next day, I asked the general manager of the hotel to please have housekeepers who speak English clean my room because I cannot communicate with non-English speakers. She became defensive. She explained that they all spoke English, that she did not discriminate in hiring, and that the housekeeper understood what I said but that I had "startled" her.

The next time I requested a housekeeper, a front desk employee and the housekeeper came to my room. I told the front desk employee what I needed. She then spoke into her phone, which translated her words from English into Spanish.

I was asked to check out of the hotel the following day. It was then that I told the employee at the front desk that I have autism. I was embarrassed to tell him, but after I did, the management relented and allowed me to remain in the hotel.

I did not feel I had done anything wrong. Somewhere in the communication between the housekeeper, the general manager, and myself, there was a problem. My therapist said it could have been my tone of voice, posture, etc. Honestly, I do not know what I did wrong, if anything. The DSM-5 says that autistics may use "inappropriate approaches that seem aggressive or disruptive."[4] For me, this incident was just another miscommunication in a long line of miscommunications. It happens to me all the time.

* * *

During large-scale family events at my mother and stepfather's house, rather than sit with family members and my mother's friends, I would try to spend the entire time upstairs in my bedroom with the door closed. These family events occurred when I was approximately 30 to 50 years of age. I would be quiet in my bedroom without experiencing any stress until my mother demanded I go downstairs and spend time with family and her guests. To keep her happy, I would socialize for 10 to 15 minutes each hour and spend the rest of the time upstairs. That pattern continued for as long as the party lasted.

Those at the party would be somewhat satisfied that they'd seen me, and I felt better than I would have if I'd been forced to remain downstairs for multiple hours at a time.

My mother never understood why I wanted to be alone during her parties. After all, they were my family and my mother's friends whom I'd known for decades. Why would I want to be alone? I needed to be alone because I hate small talk and the questions I would have to answer. I was also uncomfortable with the noise and the number of people in the house.

I recall a saying about being more alone in a crowd than when a person is by himself. I cannot explain exactly why this occurs. I feel intensely isolated in a crowd, very separate from the group, especially at parties. Many people who do not have autism prefer the social aspects of being with others. I could never understand that. I am happiest being alone with my thoughts.

The problem is bridging these two different views. The person with autism usually wants to be left alone, while the neurotypical often craves interaction. It is oftentimes difficult to connect between the two groups. **By attempting to understand the issues facing those on the autism spectrum, neurotypicals will have an easier time empathizing and compromising with us.**

I have a friend who had a young son on the autism spectrum. His son didn't say hello to everyone when he walked into a room full of people. I was trying to avoid the crowd myself when I heard his mother punish the boy by taking away his electronics. All the boy heard was that he was being punished for something he didn't understand. His mother believed her son was breaking social norms and that he should inherently understand those rules.

After his mother punished her son by taking away his electronics, his father tried to soften the situation by tickling him. This is a behavior many autistics hate: unwanted touch.

Later that afternoon, I explained to the father that his son was in his own world. He didn't have the flexibility to always be social when his parents wanted him to be. I told him I dealt with parties at my mother's house by hiding upstairs and separating myself from the group most of the time. After this conversation, the father seemed to better understand his son's situation.

By understanding the issues their children are experiencing, neurotypical parents can explain to their children how they should act in social environments and stop being upset with them because they don't instinctually understand the world the same way neurotypicals do.

How can the two groups come together? The biggest change will occur when each side moves as close to the center as they can. Some days, it might be possible for us to interact more. Other days, we may hide under our blankets waiting for the crowd to go home. Because of their life experiences, older persons with autism have a better sense of what is socially acceptable and generally can move to the center more easily than autistic children can.

However, this advance still may not be far enough for those not on the spectrum. It's my hope that neurotypicals can be patient enough to let us, no matter our age, slowly emerge – as far as we are able – from our communication box. If those on the spectrum can take only a few steps toward the center, please meet us as far as we can go, even if it is nowhere near the center.

Chapter 2

Why Are Relationships So Difficult to Build?

I often feel it would be easier to build a pyramid than it is for a person on the autism spectrum to have a relationship with another person. After all, having a meaningful, loving relationship is a challenge that requires all the resources an autistic person does not have in abundance: communication, flexibility, and seeing the world from the other person's point of view.

Some people with autism are happiest being alone in life because it is easier, less stressful, and less frustrating. Others, like myself, have longed for many decades to find a person to love who can respect them despite their uniqueness.

As challenging as it is for two neurotypicals to form a long-lasting relationship, it is much more difficult to build one between a person on the spectrum and a neurotypical. Relationships can and do form, but only with much effort from both groups.

Unfortunately, the divorce rate between couples when one person is on the autism spectrum is approximately 80 percent.[5] This chapter can help reduce communication difficulties for couples who are dating and married couples. And, hopefully, lower the divorce rate.

It's time to break out of your no relationship or failed relationship box.

* * *

At what point in the relationship should an autistic tell a neurotypical they have autism? First, listen to your "gut feelings." They will always guide you in the right direction. Second, tell the other person when the relationship has had a chance to deepen, not on your early dates. Neurotypicals often begin relationships slowly. Third, when the other person speaks about their personal issue(s), that could be a good time to tell them that you are on the autism spectrum. Again, listen to your gut. Fourth, to prevent a problem in a relationship that is caused by autism, share with them that you are autistic. For example, if the other person wants to go to a concert, but you have difficulty dealing with noise, you'll probably want to explain that because you are on the autism spectrum, loud noises upset you. It is entirely up to you if you tell the other person you have autism.

If you are having a challenge during a business transaction or social interaction, it is important to share with the other person as soon as you can that you are autistic. As mentioned in Chapter 1, my opening up enabled me to remain in the hotel after the general manager asked me to leave.

* * *

There are three primary challenges for those of us on the spectrum:

1. Communication
2. Flexibility
3. Ability to see things from the other person's perspective

Communication is the first obstacle. Those with autism do not understand subtext, the real meaning behind words. We generally understand only the literal words that are spoken, not the message the speaker may really be trying to get across. For example, say you ask a friend how they are doing and they say "fine," when they are not OK. An autistic person would take them at their word that they are not having a problem. We don't notice signs of stress or anger like crossed arms, biting a lip, or a raised voice.

Sometimes subtext is used to avoid hurting someone; other times it is just a general communication tool. If you have autism, the subtext used by a neurotypical only causes confusion. We are often left wondering why people cloak what they really mean with subtext. We find it baffling. If you, as an autistic person, find yourself in this situation, clarify what neurotypicals are trying to get across by asking for an explanation.

Subtext is very difficult for an autistic to learn. It takes many years of practice, often decades. Even then, we will catch only a minute amount of deeper meaning behind the words.

I was speaking with a professor's secretary on the telephone when she asked, "Do you have a reason to call?" I laughed and said, "Of course I have a reason to call. Why else would I be calling?" I later figured out that she was trying to ask WHY I wanted to talk to her boss. He never returned my call.

Most communication is nonverbal. While I was in high school, my mother would always say that I didn't hear her unless she was screaming at me. I did not notice her nonverbal communication, so she became frustrated and would scream. I still miss most nonverbal communication.

Besides subtext, we miss tone of voice. Not only do we have a problem interpreting the tone of voice of someone speaking to us but also interpreting our own tone of voice when we speak to others. Lately, I have been struggling with that challenge. Others think I am angry when I am not angry at all; I am only trying to explain a situation. Those on the spectrum need to listen to their tone of voice when they speak.

By the time a person on the spectrum is old enough to be married, hopefully that person will have had years of therapy behind them to help teach them about their communications missteps. Once we are made aware of how to act in a particular situation, we have the ability to alter our behavior. Change takes time; it is not immediate.

Information sinks in better with some autistics via written messages. Non-autistics can experiment with both speaking and writing. This will help you gauge which is more effective for a particular person on the spectrum.

If you are neurotypical, tell those with autism WHAT you need in a very straightforward manner. If they still do not understand, explain WHY you need something done in a certain way, at a certain time, etc.

To help your partner communicate with you, not only should you verbally tell them and/or write down your needs, but also explain how you FEEL about the situation and how your partner can best fulfill your needs. Those on the spectrum ***need a detailed roadmap.***

Rather than saying, "We need to talk more," consider guiding. Say something like: "I feel very alone when you go to the other side of the house and play on your Xbox for five hours after dinner. I want us to sit down every night for one hour after we eat and talk about what happened in our workplaces and how we feel about it. When we talk about our feelings, I know that you really care about me."

Those on the autism spectrum cannot read body language. In an autism group I belong to, we watched a video about body language. Not one person in the group could pick up the subtleties. We also are unable to share our feelings with others via body language. I am told that my face is "expressionless." Others have no idea if I am happy, sad, or upset. They have to ask me.

It may also be very helpful to find a therapist who has experience working with people on the autism spectrum. Sessions can be completed individually and as a couple. I recommend that both partners talk with the therapist alone, and then together with the therapist.

I began seeing my most recent therapist shortly after I began working in Phoenix in 2005. We both feel that I have made a great deal of progress in how I communicate with others. Because of my forward movement, I now talk with her a few times a year rather than every two weeks.

Do not expect your autistic partner to move as far as you would like when it comes to communication. You need to veer away from the desire for your partner to *always* be able to tell you their feelings. Perhaps that is no different from what neurotypical couples experience.

Persons with autism communicate to transfer information, not for interpersonal connection. We don't chitchat. When we talk, often it is to communicate about a favorite topic which we know very, very well. My expertise is in investments. I spend hours everyday reading on the internet about what is going on in the national economy. Most of the time, the stock markets make perfect sense to me. I also keep up with national and international politics and the weather because those things affect my investments. I can turn any conversation toward investing. Others on the spectrum may love to talk about trains, Star

Trek, or computers.

Flexibility is the second obstacle and can be another deal-breaker between a couple. Years ago, I made plans with my girlfriend to go somewhere during the week. At the last moment, she canceled our date because she hadn't finished her college assignments. Most guys would have taken the change in stride. I didn't. Autistics generally have difficulty with last-minute changes. I made a big fuss about it, which caused her to become very upset for days.

Relationships are all about give-and-take, going with the flow, sharing your feelings with your significant other, and trying new things because the other person wants to keep the relationship fresh. These are obstacles that are difficult for autistics to surmount. For the sake of the relationship, **those on the spectrum must think about the other person's needs.** If we don't work on this as hard as we can, our partner will eventually give up and leave. A neurotypical will likely get bored going to the same place or same restaurant every time they go out with someone on the autism spectrum. Autistics may resist at first but find they enjoy the art museum or whatever new activities their partner wants to engage in. But they need help easing into new things. Meanwhile, they must remember that **refusing to compromise is not an option.**

A story I was told teaches that it is better to be like a tree that bends in the face of high winds than a tree that cannot bend and then breaks in two during bad weather. Be flexible, not rigid.

Here's an example of a time I did well being flexible, mastering give-and-take, and understanding subtext. I live near Phoenix, Arizona, home to a world-famous Native American museum. A few years ago, I attended the Heard Museum Guild Indian Fair and Market with a female friend. This is my favorite annual event in Phoenix. Approximately 600 Native American artists present their jewelry, pottery, paintings, baskets, etc. The fair was scheduled to close at 5 p.m. At 3:45 p.m., my friend asked if I was ready to leave. Two things went through in my mind. First, I did not want to leave until the event ended at 5. Second, I knew my friend had work to finish at home that was making her anxious. If I hadn't known she had a busy schedule, I would have told her I was not ready to leave. She wasn't really asking me if I wanted to leave. She was saying in a very nice way that SHE wanted to leave. I went with the flow and said, "Sure, let's go." In this instance, I was able to put her feelings ahead of my desire.

Flexibility goes hand-in-hand with change. As mentioned earlier, this is not one of our strong suits. Autistics must have consistency. We cling to it because we have learned to navigate a small section of the outside world, which brings us comfort. Change brings new obstacles and new challenges, which we struggle to understand. We are beginning anew when there is an unfamiliar change.

Most people on the autism spectrum do the same things again and again because it is what we know, and the repetition makes us feel more secure. For example, I eat cereal with water (yes, with water) everyday. Breakfast does not feel right if I eat anything other than cereal with water. I get takeout at the same restaurants and always order the same food, listen to the same music all the time, and overall, don't take too many chances in life (except, of course, writing this book!). If we want relationships, autistics have to learn to be less rigid and more expansive.

Because the world is changing – constantly – we must realize that we will have to change too, at least some of the time.

Seeing the world from the other person's perspective is the third obstacle. If you are having difficulty communicating with a neurotypical, try looking at the world from the other person's point of view. Look at yourself from their eyes. Are you being reasonable? Afraid? Stubborn for no reason?

Sometimes I ask a friend, or my therapist, what they think about something I am considering. When a trusted confidant, or several persons, tell me I am wrong, I am wise to listen to – and follow – their suggestions. My grandmother on my mother's side of my family used to tell my mother that "seven can't be wrong and one right." Meaning that my mother's parents, brother, and sisters couldn't all agree and be wrong, when my mother was the only person who thought another way and believed she was right.

* * *

There also are three things that can destroy a relationship for those of us on the spectrum:

1. Not looking your partner in their eyes

2. Too much honesty
3. Anger or frustration when we miss subtext

If you are on the autism spectrum, take these three thoughts to heart because your relationship may be in danger if you don't (unless you are romantically connected with another autistic): First, look at the person you are having a conversation with, at least occasionally. I know it is incredibly difficult to concentrate and think when looking at another person. I am in the same boat. But, if you want to connect with someone else and remain with them for the long-term, you have to look at them from time to time, even briefly. A woman I know who was living with a person she believed was autistic told me it "drove her crazy" that her live-in boyfriend wouldn't look at her while she was talking to him.

Neurotypicals require eye contact. Without it, they assume that autistics are not listening to them, don't care, and/or are blowing them off. That is not what is happening in an autistic's mind. Personally, I can usually concentrate much better if I am not looking at someone. I cannot focus on my thoughts when I am looking at someone while I am talking or when they are speaking. Try to meet in the middle. Tell your neurotypical partner that you can't focus on what they are saying if you are always looking at them, but you will try to look into their eyes for a short time. A second option is to look at the other person's forehead for a moment. This way, they will think you are looking at them and you can maintain your concentration more easily than actually looking into their eyes. If you won't make the effort to move closer to what your partner needs in this area, you will likely have serious problems in your relationship. For neurotypicals, having their partner look at them is important.

The second problem that can destroy a relationship is too much honesty, or as a neurotypical would describe it, thoughtlessness or cruelty. Yes, autistics require honesty. We are almost always honest, and we expect our friend or partner to be honest, too. Lying clouds communication. This goes back to subtext. **We need directness and we expect honesty.** Lying, even a "white lie," is exactly the opposite of honesty, and it breaks trust with us. We want total honesty, but that is not always what people who are not on the spectrum want. For example, they don't consider a white lie dishonest if they are using it in attempt to keep the peace.

Total honesty can appear mean to a neurotypical. For example, when a friend asked me if she was as fat as another person in the room, I was thinking, "Yep, you sure are!" After years of therapy and striving to understand how neurotypicals think and behave, I realized that if I had been honest with her, she would have been very upset with me. I said, "No." **Just because you think or feel something does not mean you have to say it.** Use discretion. Before you speak, think of how your words might affect the other person.

"White lies" are not only OK, but preferable, in the neurotypical world if you do not want to hurt the other person's feelings. It is essential to think about the other person's feelings now, or they won't be around later.

Third, don't be angry when an autistic misses subtext. It is only on a rare occasion that we will catch it. Those without autism believe they communicated information non-verbally to an autistic. Unfortunately, we very scarcely pick up subtext.

* * *

How can a neurotypical begin, or strengthen, a relationship with a person on the spectrum? Again, explain in detail what you want and need. Here's an example: rather than saying, "Let's go out to eat," be more detailed. Instead, say something like, "How about at 7 p.m. on Saturday, let's have dinner at Tottie's Asian Fusion 2?" Or say, "Let's stay home and watch my favorite TV show, *Heartland*." Autistics will understand what you are looking for when you share with us exactly what you want.

A second way to strengthen a relationship is to be understanding if an autistic doesn't understand everything that a neurotypical says the first time around. One suggestion is to repeat a second time the things you really want us to know or understand. Better yet, write a note on a piece of paper or send an e-mail or text. Autistics think more clearly when communication is in writing than when it's oral.

Constructing a pyramid has both backbreaking and mental challenges. It is difficult work. One major miscue and the pyramid will be lost. For those attempting to build a lasting relationship, focus more on the other person and less on yourself. Let your non-autistic partner know that you do not understand subtext. Communication and thoughtfulness can win you a partner. Being rigid and stubborn will cause your connection to break.

Chapter 3

Dreams and Aspirations

Without dreams, we live our lives aimlessly. It is as if we are walking through a forest without a compass. Dreams take us to a magical place, a destination that is waiting for us. This place is our goal(s). Our souls cheer when we reach our goals, and they cry in desperation when we don't even try.

There are no insignificant dreams.

I always remind myself of a brilliant thought, which is a variation of an Oscar Wilde quote, If you reach for the stars you won't get stuck in the mud.

Without dreams, without goals, we live a colorless, monotone life.

Your dream may be to help feed the homeless people in your community, to write a book, to travel, to help patrons at your local library, to make jewelry, to find a job fixing computers, or any of myriad other possibilities. Dreams are endless, like the stars in the sky. Pick one or more and use them as guiding lights in your life.

Many people with autism have had their dreams crushed throughout their lives by well-meaning parents, teachers, and coworkers, as well as bullies.

Numerous people tell us we cannot succeed at work, find a lifelong partner, or even have friends. We consistently hear the same old mantra: "You cannot do, you cannot have, you cannot be. You are different."

Most anyone who is told constantly that they will fail WILL FAIL. Alternately, if they are frequently reminded how capable they are, they

WILL SUCCEED. Words can encourage or discourage. The person who hears your words – particularly those that are repeated again and again – will become what you say, whether your words are positive or negative. This phenomenon is called the Pygmalion Effect. Having someone who supports us can make all the difference in reaching our dreams.

In the late 1980s, I shared a dream of mine with my mother and stepfather. I wanted to open a religious newspaper in Des Moines. My stepfather ran his own printing business, so he had an understanding of how extremely difficult it is to start a business from scratch. My experience at the time was as a reporter, editor and photographer for weekly and daily newspapers. My stepfather told me that starting a newspaper would not work, so I didn't even attempt to fulfill my dream. Maybe it would have worked, maybe not. I will never know because I did not even try.

The first step toward reaching your dreams is encouragement from yourself and others; this is key, both verbally and in thought. Why in thought? If you believe you (or another person) can reach a goal, that will influence your (or their) actions. Also, subconsciously the other person will pick up that you believe in them, thus giving them added support.

Walking hand-in-hand with encouragement is hope. Having a dream without believing you will succeed is like trying to drive a car to your destination with an empty fuel tank. Hope is the figurative fuel that moves us toward our goals.

Personally, my main dream has always been to help others. I have done so by volunteering since high school; working as a newspaper reporter so I could share information with the public and make people feel better about their lives; and, publishing this book. My most difficult challenge was publishing this book. It took me nine years of writing and rewriting before it was published.

The next step after encouragement and hope is constructing a plan. **Plans are the ladders that will allow you to reach your dreams.** Some plans are detailed, others are not. Write down your plan and then review it as often as you need to. Completing parts of the plan to accomplish your dreams will serve as internal encouragement. Let yourself feel good when you reach each step on the path to your dreams – it is something to be proud of!

If, after much effort, you are unable to reach your dreams, do not despair. You surely experienced successes along the way that you would not have had if you never even tried. Because you stretched beyond your old abilities, you have become a new and better person. When you try your best and give it your all, you are a winner.

Your dreams are in the stars. Look up. Dream big. Work hard to transform your life into what you want it to be.

Chapter 4

Positivity Despite Life-Altering Diseases

I was introduced to Heather Olsen, an energy healer with psychic and medium abilities, who lives in Pennsylvania, by my excellent St. Louis Doctor of Osteopath, Rajiv Yadava.

Before I met Heather, I had been in a very dark place since at least high school, when I constantly thought about killing myself. I have only had peace and contentment twice in my life: the summer before I began a reporting position in a small Missouri town and after I completed one year of work at the same job. A decade before that time, and decades following, I dealt with deep, dark problems, one after another.

Heather and I met over the phone in October 2014. She said that I was "very, very, very sad and had no self-esteem." She described me as feeling like everyone was against me, betraying me, and lying to me, when I interviewed her for this book. She also reminded me that I had been angry at the world. Heather showed me how to look at situations from different angles. She described what she did as tapping into my past and helping me release my traumas. She said she also "used energy work and intuition to get to the core of my self-esteem issues" and she "worked on clearing my past emotional issues that were the core causes of my physical ailments."

She said that "everything" has changed about me since we met. I try to live my best life, I see the silver lining in dark clouds, I have come out of my comfort zone, and I even tell jokes now.

If I had not met Heather, I might not be alive today because I needed a great deal of positivity to get through three serious diseases.

My first major disease was Hereditary Spastic Paraplegia (HSP), which causes weakness and stiffness in my legs. Many people who have this disease use canes, walkers, or wheelchairs. HSP has caused balance issues for me and extreme pain in my feet while walking or sitting. The further I walk, the more pain I feel in my feet. Without wearing gauntlet braces, I would not be able to walk for long periods. Around 2010, when my current podiatrist examined me for the first time, she thought I would be in a wheelchair one or two years later. To her surprise, I can still walk. HSP is rare, and there is no cure.

Chronic Inflammatory Demyelinating Polyneuropathy (CIDP) is the second physical problem I have. It causes weakness in my legs and extreme body fatigue. My myelin sheaths (fatty, insulating layers that surround the nerve fibers) are damaged. Because of this illness, I have neuropathy in my feet, which sometimes spreads to my fingers and arms. An antibody drug I used to receive every three or four years but now take 12 times a year removes the neuropathy from my fingers, arms, and right foot for a period of time. Unfortunately, neuropathy in my left foot does not dissipate. CIDP also is rare and has no cure.

Lastly, I also have Waldenstrom's Macroglobulinemia (WM). WM is a blood cancer that also causes neuropathy in my hands and feet, as well as fatigue. It is another rare disease that cannot be cured. I once heard a Mayo Clinic doctor say that if a person contracts cancer, this is the best one to have. Approximately 1,100 to 1,500 persons in the United States develop WM each year. Heather told me six months before I had any symptoms that she could sense there was a problem with my blood.

Besides these three major diseases I struggle with Obsessive Compulsive Disorder (OCD). The more stress I experience, the worse my OCD, although I have far fewer rituals now compared to when I was in college. OCD blocked me from completing my master's degree. It still dramatically slows down my reading and enjoyment of books, and it has created obstacles in writing this book.

Looking at my life in a positive manner has made it easier to deal daily with my numerous disabilities. I have been able to maintain an optimistic attitude because I remind myself that everything happens in this world for a reason, although we may or may not find out why in our lifetime. There could be an unlimited number of reasons why an event might happen: it could be because of what occurred in your past life, what you have done in this life, or what you may do in a future life. Additionally, what initially appears to be a negative event might wind up saving you from a much worse episode. Be happy about that. What you believe is a sad event may, in the long run, not be sad at all.

I met Heather so I could alter my perspective from a very negative one to a positive one. That transformation has allowed me to hurdle over my medical difficulties, write this book, and experience other favorable effects in this world. She helped me realize that the events in my past were not my fault, and I should not blame myself for them. That is why, over time, I have been able to adopt a happier focus.

If you're in a negative place right now, my suggestion is that you be grateful for who you are, what has happened in your life, and for everything you have. What can bring your life to a happier level is writing in a gratitude journal. Write each day what makes you happy. On days when you are sad, your previous writing will make you happier. You probably have much more to be thankful for than you realize.

Chapter 5

Surrounded by Bullies

People on any level of the autism spectrum are constantly harassed by bullies because we are very different from neurotypicals. I have experienced this challenge all my life.

In elementary school, I was teased and isolated from others. Having few friends, I learned to live in my own world. What I mean by that is that I lived in my head, not in the outside world with others. This pattern became a safety mechanism. If I had not isolated myself mentally, I either would have killed myself due to the constant stress or seriously lashed out in a dangerous way at those who constantly harassed me.

My major challenges began in junior high school. I was constantly bullied in seventh and eighth grades, and less so in ninth grade. Every day, it was the same ol' thing – only the people would change. From the moment I waited at the bus stop until I got home, I was constantly teased, harassed, and bullied. Going to school was hell on Earth. One day in my seventh grade gym class, I was in three separate fights. Mind you, I have never started a fight to this day, yet I was forced to fight to defend myself.

I was bullied occasionally in ninth grade, but I was generally harassed less. I believe this is because I had been tough enough physically and mentally to stick with my junior high school wrestling team the entire season, while some of the bullies dropped out after just a few days. I was also bullied less often because the older kids who had given me such a difficult time moved on to high school.

Fortunately, in tenth and eleventh grades, I had a few friends who also happened to be outcasts. We formed a nerdy clique that no one else wanted to join. This group allowed me some sanity, or normality, in my life. We ate lunch together and hung out after school, playing tennis or ping pong or going to movies.

My mother knew I was having extreme difficulty fitting in at school, yet I felt as if she blamed me for my problems. When I was in high school, my sister was beaten up (she never started a fight, either) by a girl with a baton. Immediately afterward, we built a house and moved to a different school district for my senior year. I knew only a few people at the new school when I began my last year of high school. I studied hard and kept to myself. I never understood why I had to go through hell for seventh and eighth grades, but our family moved as soon as my sister had difficulty just once.

* * *

Unfortunately, the bullying began again in college. I had major problems in my dorm. In my sophomore year, the University of Missouri-Columbia paired me with a roommate who drank heavily every weekend. I rarely drank in college, and when I did, it was a very small amount. As you might have guessed, my roommate and I didn't get along. After a month or two, he moved out, but he came back to my dorm floor every once in a while to enlist others against me. After he moved out, I would find myself "pennied" (when someone on the outside of the door wedges pennies above the deadbolt to keep the door from opening) into my dorm room. One night, after I walked out of the shower, I found shaving cream covering the entire door of my dorm room.

The scariest incident occurred in my sophomore year while sleeping in my room. I suddenly woke up in the dark to find someone hovering over me. He ran out of the room and into the bathroom where I found him standing next to the urinal peeing. I should have clobbered him, but I didn't touch him. Not until I wrote this paragraph did I ever think about or realize what he'd been planning to do: pee on me.

In some ways, what happened with my roommate when I was a freshman, who was a black student, was more shocking, especially since I thought we were getting along well. He was a junior preparing to enter law school. He introduced me to jazz, constantly talked to me, and took me out grocery shopping with him off-campus. One of his previous roommates had put tape across the middle of the floor and told him he was not allowed to cross the line to the other side of the room. Even in the late '70s, black students were not always accepted on campus.

In the middle of the second semester, I found a crumpled piece of paper on the floor next to the trash can. I opened it and read it because I thought it had fallen off my desk. My roommate had written that he wanted to move. He became defensive when I asked him about it. He eventually explained that he'd changed his mind about moving, because he knew I would have had an even more difficult time with a new roommate, which turned out to be a correct assessment of what occurred in my sophomore year. My roommate never explained, and I never understood what I did wrong or why he wanted to move out.

Looking back at my college days at Mizzou, I realize I was part of the problem. I was noticed for all the wrong reasons. At the beginning of my freshman year, I would take bread from the cafeteria and feed the birds in front of the huge cafeteria windows where many of my fellow students could see me. Soon after I began feeding my two-winged friends, I became known as "Bird Man." I didn't know this was a problem until my roommate kindly informed me. In college, I often was still in my own world and didn't consider the problems being alone would cause me.

College was challenging enough without being picked on and having disabilities that severely affected my academic experience. I was viewed as different and strange because of autism; I didn't know how to live without being negatively noticed by others.

As in tenth and eleventh grades, I was lucky to find a few friends in college. An acquaintance I met in the Boy Scouts, who was four years older than I, introduced me to a group of guys. Paul Kirkman and the rest of my posse of friends kept me mentally stimulated and at times took me out of my box into the external world. We ate dinner together, debated every issue under the sun, and hung out seven days a week.

* * *

Bullying does not end when an autistic graduates from high school or college. At a job I started when I was 34, I was constantly harassed by a few of my coworkers. One time, they passed along a note to everyone – including my two supervisors – making fun of me. The bullies then put the note in my workplace mailbox so I would feel terrible.

In another position, when I was 45, my supervisor's assistant worked with me one morning. Afterward, she told me she had previously been afraid to talk to me, but realized after our session that I was a nice person. She didn't explain why she had been afraid to speak to me.

Failure to be accepted is a constant problem for many of us. What can we do to improve the situation? Autistics do not like to chitchat the way neurotypicals do. They talk about the weather, the local sports teams, movies, or ask what the other person did over the weekend. Those things are uninteresting to most autistic people.

But I have to remind myself not to go on and on about my favorite topics. I could talk forever about the stock market or politics, though this is unacceptable to most everyone. As difficult as it might be, if you're an autistic trying to fit into the neurotypical world, try to be as breezy and light as you can with your conversations.

As mentioned in Chapter 2, autistics rarely look at the person we are speaking to because we have difficulty thinking and looking at someone at the same time. Those without autism do not have that challenge. Quite often, if we do not look at the other person, they believe we are blowing them off or not taking them seriously. To avoid this problem, try looking at their forehead for a few moments while talking to them. That will help to keep them cheerful. If necessary, tell the neurotypical that you have autism and cannot look at and speak to them at the same time. This might go a long way toward helping them understand our difficulty with this issue.

We can improve communication with those not on the autism spectrum, but I don't believe that we can solve it completely because we are very different from them. Most of us on the spectrum want to get along with others, but some of us have no desire or capability to change how we communicate. Personally, I can make a few alterations at a time, but if I try to become a totally different person I will be overwhelmed. Plus, who wants to change everything about themselves, whether they're autistic or neurotypical? A few neurotypicals will bring us into their world; others will not. Because we stand out from others, it's been my experience that we will likely always be bullied to a certain extent, or remain unaccepted as individuals.

I continue to try to break out of my communication box and, as a result, to experience less bullying. This has resulted in a better understanding about how to communicate better with others and the realization that I am judged by what I say and do.

Chapter 6

Employment

Most of us desire independence, to be on our own, to live life our way. It takes money to be the captain of our ship. Bringing in money through work can allow each of us to steer our life in the direction we desire to go.

For many people, being at work is a thoughtless exercise. They have to be there to support their family and do what society expects of an adult. If possible, they tie employment to their dreams. They have a vision of themselves and the way they want to help make the world a better place. With that type of mindset, employment rises above daily drudgery; it connects you to your higher self and forges your dreams.

Sometimes it is not possible to tie employment to your dreams. If your work is not directly tied to fulfilling your dreams, perhaps you can focus on them outside of work, on something like creating art, for example. If you are fortunate, you might be able to merge your employment and your dreams at some point in the future. Be gentle with yourself if this doesn't appear to be possible for you.

"Special interests may be a source of pleasure and motivation and provide avenues for education and employment later in life," according to DSM-5.[6]

Please remember that the range of disabilities on the autism spectrum is quite wide. Some people can live on their own, while others cannot. Some can control their emotions better than others. Some speak quite loudly, while others are sensitive to loud noises. Some have issues with certain kinds of light. Because the range is expansive, it can affect both how long it might take for an autistic person to be hired and their ability to retain a position.

People on the spectrum have great difficulty getting hired and keeping the jobs they get. The unemployment rate has been reported to be between 75 to 85 percent for those with autism.[7] I believe our lack of communication skills both during the interview process and while on the job contributes greatly to our incredibly high unemployment rate.

It's time to break out of your unemployment box.

While looking for a position, ask yourself: "Do I have the skills to be hired for this position, or must I learn how to do the job?" Perhaps the skills you have not picked up in school can be developed with an internship. Internships come in both paid and unpaid varieties.

If you are in high school, talk with your guidance counselor about the possibility of an internship. College students can reach out to teachers, department heads, and their college's Career Services Department. The CSD should have a list of companies offering internships, along with the responsibilities and number of hours per week particular internships require. You can also visit a company's website to see if an internship might be available. If no information is listed on the website, send an e-mail or call the company or organization's human resources department.

Remember that the company's secretary is your gateway to influential people inside the business. What the secretary thinks of you is more important than you realize. If you are friendly and businesslike, there is a greater chance you will be put through to the person who can help you. When you are interviewing for an internship (or a job), it is not uncommon for the decision-maker to ask the secretary what they think of you.

If you are offered an internship, think of it as a "real" job, whether it is a paid or unpaid position. Act businesslike at all times and dress appropriately for the position. This is your opportunity to shine. Learn as much as you can while interning and do what you can to become part of the team. Focus on remaining flexible. On occasion, the internship may lead to a job with that company. If you succeed at your internship, there's a very good chance you will pick up a solid work reference, which is quite important.

If an internship in your area of interest is not available, consider volunteering for an organization that can use your skills. These positions are varied and numerous. You can find them in hospitals, libraries, nonprofits, etc. Find one or two (to give yourself some variety) that are tailored to your job interests. For example, if you want to become a computer programmer but there are no internships available in a for-profit company, perhaps your local library has a position for a volunteer to help the staff with their computer system. Or, if you would like to learn how to write grants, many nonprofit organizations would appreciate your assistance. You can get on-the-job training in grant-writing, and they will pick up an eager volunteer (you!).

Internships and volunteer positions can also help you determine if you are really interested in a particular job or field before you invest a great deal of time and money on a degree program at a college or university.

The skills you pick up while volunteering are just as relevant as if you learned them from an internship or a paid job, but there will likely be less stress, more fun, and greater flexibility.

Just like an internship, volunteering can lead to a job offer. It can also earn you a work reference.

I have volunteered with numerous organizations. The work ranged from writing news releases and feature articles to event photography for the Alzheimer's Association Greater Missouri Chapter in St. Louis. I also spent time contacting organizations around the world to procure publications for the Billie Jane Baguley Library and Archives at the Heard Museum in Phoenix and served food to seniors as part of a religious youth group in high school.

While volunteering for the Alzheimer's Association, I helped the organization and my community, increased my skills (this opportunity would have been perfect for a newbie), and kept my name in the public eye, which was important, as I also owned a writing, photography, and PR company at the time.

Besides volunteering, I had an internship working as an Ombudsman in the Lieutenant Governor's office in the State of Missouri. I helped solve citizens' state governmental problems.

* * *

People with autism have multiple challenges, among them networking and making contact with others. Most open positions are not listed on internet job boards, websites, or in newspapers; they are uncovered through professional and personal networks. You must gather the strength and courage to meet others through professional organizations, alumni groups, and/or networking events. Your contacts also include friends in your field of interest and those you meet while working as an intern, a volunteer, or in a job.

Networking is a give-and-take process. Not only are you making connections with others for your benefit, but they are looking at the business relationship both to help you and for assistance from you to help them, now and in the future. Remember, not everything is about you.

Networking is a skill you must hone by practicing often. It can be very difficult for someone on the autism spectrum because it involves strong communication skills. Educators and counselors can teach us how to communicate more effectively. Personally, I am better today than I was decades ago, but I am still not good or comfortable with it.

Numerous books explain the ins-and-outs of being a competent networker. An excellent book on this subject, and employment overall, for those with autism is titled, *The Complete Guide to Getting a Job for People with Asperger's Syndrome: Find the Right Career and Get Hired*, by Barbara Bissonnette. She takes the reader step-by-step from finding the right career to resume writing, networking, the pluses and minuses of asking for an accommodation, etc. I found the publication very helpful in untangling many of my problem areas, including interviewing.

Improving our communication skills a few steps beyond where they currently are will definitely help in getting hired and staying employed.

As mentioned on page 15, looking at a person while talking to them face-to-face is very important to a neurotypical. I know how difficult it is to think while looking and talking to a person, but if you can do it for even a short amount of time, it will help a lot, both while networking and during the interview process. If you can't look them in their eyes, try glancing at their forehead. Neurotypicals will think you are looking directly at them. If you do not do this, they are likely to believe you are being dishonest or just ignoring them.

Chitchatting is also important to neurotypicals, while networking and especially after you are hired. Talk to them about the weather, a good movie you just watched, or what you did over the weekend. This is how you can make connections with others. Personally, I don't like chitchatting, I would much rather talk about investments, national and international politics, or the world economy. If we want to keep our positions, we have to do at least some of what others expect.

One of the most difficult aspects of being hired full- or part-time for a person on the autism spectrum is navigating the interview process. I almost always had behavioral interviews, which focus on the past to try to predict the future. They never worked out well for me. For example, when an interviewer asks, "Tell me what you did when your supervisor criticized your work," they are looking for specific examples. No matter how much I practiced or considered possible questions beforehand, I would always get tripped up on these types of questions.

First, I was nervous about getting the job, not to mention trying to be comfortable with the interviewer(s) and trying to answer their questions in the ways that made sense to them. It was STRESS, STRESS, STRESS.

There are numerous types of job interviews you could go through. To learn about the various possibilities, use Google on your smartphone or computer and type, "What types of interviews are there?" Read about the possible situations you might find yourself in and prepare for them. By doing this, you will be as ready as possible for your interview(s). It is not easy to master interviewing, but master it we must.

On occasion, a job will be offered. Then comes the biggest challenge: the job itself.

Succeeding in an interview is stressful enough for me; trying to keep a job is 100 steps beyond that. The job offer comes in, and then worry takes over because I know it is difficult to meet the employer's standards. I become internally upset when a supervisor points out a mistake or when I cannot get along with those around me.

The potholes are many and the risks are high. **First pothole: Getting along with others.**

No matter how illustrious your work, you must be accepted by most of the people you are working with. This is more important than anything else on the job. Try to smile and be friendly. Again, neurotypicals for the most part believe that chitchatting is important. For me, chitchatting is incredibly difficult, especially in group situations. Even so, small talk forges relationships and friendships, which bring us to **Teamwork**.

Nearly all positions require working with others, be it taking orders at McDonald's, working in a retail store, or saving lives in a hospital.

If you are unable to get along with your team members and work toward the same goals, the company's project will either fail or be less successful than it could be. Why let the ship sink when you can keep it afloat by becoming a team player?

An issue related to teamwork is **Listening**.

Nearly everyone wants to be respected. One of the best ways to improve communication and foster teamwork is to listen. You will not have all the answers, no matter how much smarter you think you are than the rest of the team. The smallest suggestion can make the difference between success and failure. *There are several locks on the door of success. Every person on your team has one of the keys.* What this means is that everyone, including you, has the ability to fix a problem. Don't be rigid. Allow everyone's ideas to flow.

Set a goal to **do your best**.

Have an internal fire to perform at your very best. For you to move ahead in the organization, or perhaps just to keep your position, and for the team to meet its goals, you must give it your all every day. Bad days happen, of course. Mistakes occur. Don't linger over them. Don't blame others. Fix what you can and be sure you understand why the error occurred and what you can do so it doesn't happen again. No one is perfect. All anyone can ask is that you perform to the best of your ability.

These four thoughts are not only for those who are employed, have an internship, or a volunteer position, but for life in general.

* * *

You may wish to tell your employer that you have autism; this is entirely your choice. I believe that your employer will treat you better if you share with them that you are on the spectrum as soon as you are hired. There are positive and negative aspects of sharing your condition with your employer. Some employers may not hire you if you tell them during the interview process. Other employers may ask you why you didn't tell them while you were being interviewed. Do what you feel is right. If you wait until you are on the verge of losing your job, opening up *might* help you keep your position.

We must learn to tell others that we are autistic, and also to advocate for the accommodations we need. At the time I had difficulty at a major company in Phoenix, I had not yet learned I was on the spectrum. If I'd had that information, I would have told my employer that I have autism and asked them to please allow me to work in a quiet area of the office. The people chatting in the row next to me while I was working on the telephone affected my thought process while talking to customers.

Employers need to recognize that autistics have difficulties those not on the autism spectrum do not have: people talking; the buzzing sound and flickering of fluorescent lights; needing literal communication, not subtext; the smell of cleaning compounds, new carpets, fragrances; and etc. Supervisors, please look for solutions with your autistic employees. What employers may feel is "normal" for everyone, could be considered discrimination by those on the autism spectrum.

Employers should also understand that those on the autism spectrum usually learn much better when they can see or physically do what is needed on the job, rather than having instructions explained verbally. If a streaming video can be made, the person could watch it several times if necessary. Another option might be to make the video available on the autistic person's cellphone.

Besides telling employers that you are on the spectrum, you may want to share with others outside of work that you have autism. As I wrote in Chapter 1, I was asked to leave a hotel. However, when I disclosed that I have autism, they allowed me to stay and were much nicer to me. Of course, I cannot promise that others will be nicer to you if you disclose, but they *should* be more understanding and flexible.

I am finding it much easier to tell others I have autism today than I did several years ago. There seems to be an understanding that this is a genetic condition I was born with. Also, it sheds light on why I act as I do. Once neurotypicals have clarity, they seem to be more empathetic.

Lately, if I know I will have to deal with others for a long period of time, I have been having my autism conversation with them early, before there is a problem, or when I feel a problem is emerging. Sharing that you are autistic may not make any difference at all to some people, but it has always worked for me.

Chapter 7

Personal Employment Challenges

In the 1980s, I worked as a staff reporter, editor, and photographer for two newspapers: the first a weekly and the second a daily publication. I was fired from both positions. My work was excellent at the weekly. I wrote features and covered numerous beats: city and county government, police and fire departments, local school board, and high school sports. If anything moved in that small town, I knew about it. For nearly 18 months, I worked seven days a week, every week, except for two. The position was difficult and demanding, but I was happy in that environment after a while. Though I nearly quit the job during my first week because I was so overwhelmed, I'm glad I toughed it out.

Two other persons were on the reporting staff: the first was an older man who slept most every afternoon at his desk; the second was a middle-aged woman who had previously taught English. The mistake I made was asking for a raise after one year on the job. I didn't realize that the owner did not want to meet with me because he did not want to pay me more. He kept saying he was too busy for us to talk. Neurotypicals would have figured out that a raise wasn't in the cards. When we did eventually meet, he showed me another small-town newspaper and said I should be doing more reporting. Mind you, the newspaper had three reporters, yet I was writing the majority of articles, taking most of the pictures, working seven days a week (the owner saw I was the only person in the office every Sunday afternoon and evening) and earning only $250 a week before taxes.

I was fired six months after the owner rejected my raise request. I believe it happened because I pushed for a meeting for more money without having the perception that the owner did not want to pay me more. Also because the owner purchased a $250,000 printing press. Two weeks after I was fired, I spoke with a friend who lived in the area who asked, "Where's the news?"

If I had known I had autism at this time, I might have been taught by a counselor about social interactions and realized I was prodding the owner for a raise he had no intention of giving me.

The daily newspaper I was working at was the second company to fire me. I do not understand why. I was told by the editor that I was "on the fast track" a few weeks after I started the job. He had a meeting with me six months later about my performance where we only talked about the upcoming company picnic. He fired me a few weeks later. What I should have done was ask for an explanation so I could either have attempted to change the editor's mind or work on the problem and perform better in my next job.

After working for both newspapers, I opened a writing, photography, and PR company in St. Louis. I had a few major successes: I won a national award for newsletters I designed, wrote and published for Missouri Goodwill Industries, and took photographs at two major events for the St. Louis Zoo. The zoo was my favorite client because of Jerry Sears, my contact there. He was incredibly creative, having won national and international awards for the zoo's newsletters, and was very kind to me. He even gave me advice about my Missouri Goodwill newsletters.

Unfortunately, after eight years I closed up shop, not because my work wasn't above par, but because I wasn't bringing in enough money.

I then worked for a large customer service company for 25 months, full-time but without benefits. Most everyone else earned benefits during their first three months on the job. I had three problems in that period: being made fun of by the other call-takers because I stuttered, lack of guidance from my supervisors, and for some unknown reason the department head refusing me benefits even though I was working 40+ hours a week.

After one week of training, I was listening to calls with an experienced call-taker. When it was time for me to take my first emergency road service call, I stuttered on the phone. The person training me laughed and immediately ran to the dispatch area to tell his friends about the incident. Shortly afterward, I became the laughingstock of the call center. Over time, most of the workers who had bullied me left the company.

Another problem was my two supervisors. When I needed assistance with a call, they would not help. They just told me to do what I wanted. I couldn't learn how to do my job well without their guidance. Sometime later, when I had a question, they would tell me that I had been there a while, so why didn't I know the answer? An older gentleman named Carl would help me from time to time, so I moved to the desk across the aisle from him. When I had a question on a call, he taught me how to handle it. That's how I learned to take emergency road service calls.

After nearly two years of putting up with harassment and not receiving the benefits I was entitled to, I finally spoke to the Human Resources Department. In response, the department head put a letter in my file threatening to fire me if my work did not improve.

One day, I walked into my work area and both my supervisors were very nice to me. That was a shock because they had always been so unpleasant to me. That day, I learned the department head had transferred to a different department within the company. A month or so later, I became full-time with benefits. I received raises and promotions for a couple of years while the new manager was on board. It was a much better working environment, and I began to train a few new hires, one-on-one, on how to take calls. My work also expanded to become a travel counselor, car and hotel reservationist, and an acting supervisor when neither supervisor was available. After two years, my first department head returned to his previous position in the call center. I still received annual raises, but no further advancements in the five years I remained on the job. I worked for this company for nearly nine years and eight months until I moved to Phoenix to help my father due to his declining health.

I think the main reason I kept my position for so long while waiting to receive benefits is that I did my very best on the job. I was an asset. Who wants to throw away a diamond? I think most people in my position would have given up and found another job. Perhaps I didn't quit because I have autism. I don't like change, no matter how rough the waters are. Or maybe it was because I have been harassed for most of my life, and I didn't know what acceptance and appreciation were.

For whatever reason, I hung on and completed more years at that job than with any other company.

I write about my job experiences to encourage you not to give up. Life is often unfair. In the long run, though, the customer service job worked out. I helped a multitude of members with situations ranging from a baby locked inside a car to offering advice on how to make a member's vacation more memorable. I also saved a lot of money, which I needed when I moved to Phoenix.

It was not until after I was no longer working for any of these companies that I learned I have autism. If I had been aware at the time that I was on the spectrum, I might have asked for and received accommodations. I believe I also might have been treated better.

Chapter 8

Managing Your Money

As mentioned in *Chapter 6: Employment*, if you desire to be the captain of your ship, you need to earn money. Beyond bringing in money, both those on the autism spectrum and neurotypicals must know how to manage their funds.

It's time to break out of the not-knowing-how-to-manage-money box.

Earning money can make you happy; knowing how to manage your money will bring you freedom and security: freedom from living with your parents, if you do not want to; the joy of taking a vacation; buying a car; purchasing electronics; and, security from losing your residence, car, etc. When you earn a living, the world opens up for you.

Additionally, when you have money, you will feel more secure from the financial bumps that everyone experiences, like unexpected car or home repairs. Most of all, having money is a protective shield from financial worry. Many people toss and turn at night while trying to sleep over concerns about how they will pay their bills. Having enough money allays those anxieties.

I have been studying money and investments for decades. Even though I am not a financial advisor, I have helped many people manage and invest their funds. I keep up with the markets daily by reading articles from CNN, CNBC, etc. For decades, I viewed the Nightly Business Report on my local public broadcasting station until it went off the air at the end of 2019. I also study Value Line (stocks) and Morningstar (mutual funds).

Too few parents and educators teach children and teenagers about finances, given what a significant difference it makes between a challenging and a comfortable financial life.

Learning how to budget your money is your first step toward becoming financially independent.

Write down on a piece of paper (I'm old school) or type on your computer your income after taxes. If you're using a computer, you might want to do this in a spreadsheet. Also, keep track of every penny you spend: rent, food, student loans, gasoline, movies, etc. Be sure to date each entry.

For example:

June 27 Grocery store $18.00
June 28 Subway restaurant $ 6.18

Yes, this is a tedious process. It will, however, tell you where you are spending your money and exactly how much you are spending. Don't be so tight that life is not enjoyable, but don't be a spendthrift either. Your goal should be to land somewhere in the middle. After a month or two, you will notice patterns in your spending. Everyone has wasteful spending. Eliminate as much of the overspending as you can.

Keep track of your spending for three months, longer if you feel it is necessary.

The second step is to bring any credit card debt to zero.

Debt is an albatross that lays on your neck like a noose. The worst kind of debt accrues via credit cards. Interest is often very high, and if you're not managing these bills or are using your credit cards frequently, it's easy for the amount to build and build, making it even more difficult to pay off what you owe. Make an effort to pay your credit card in full each month so you do not carry a balance. Most Americans owe money on their credit cards. This kind of debt is considered "bad" debt. I will write soon about the opposite, or "good" debt.

If you do have credit card debt, eliminate it by paying off your highest interest credit cards first. Let's say Credit Card A charges 17.9 percent and Credit Card B charges 13.9 percent. Work on paying off Credit Card A first because it has the highest interest rate. Don't forget to make the minimum payment on Credit Card B while you are paying off Credit Card A. When you finish paying off A, you can then use the amount of money you were spending on A to pay down B. In addition, also pay the amount you were paying as the minimum payment on B to pay down B even faster.

It is vitally important not to carry credit card debt. When you are debt-free, you will not be sucked dry from the debt itself and the corresponding interest payments. A huge worry will be off your shoulders, and your FICO score will rise. I will explain the importance of your FICO score a bit later in this chapter.

There are two types of "good" debt: car loans and mortgage loans. Unless you live in a city with a good public transportation system or you know someone who is willing to drive you to all of your destinations, you need a car. A car allows you to go everywhere, both for fun and work. You need reliable transportation to get to work. I recommend purchasing a car with payments that fit within your budget.

If you are exceptionally good at saving money, you may have accumulated enough funds for a downpayment on a condo or house. For many people, buying makes more sense than renting. Purchasing property is a topic best left to other books.

If you are lucky enough not to have any debt, congratulations! You are one of the rare persons in the United States to be debt-free.

The third step is to build an emergency fund.

In conjunction with paying down debt, build an emergency fund to help you with any emergency that may occur. This could range from tempering the blow from a loss of income if you lose your job to paying for repairs if your car breaks down, medical bills, etc. Your emergency fund will be your cushion of money that shields you from financial worry.

Many financial specialists recommend saving three to six months of expenses in your emergency fund. I think nine months is a better number for those with autism because due to our communication challenges, it can take longer for us to replace our jobs if we are laid off or fired than for someone not on the autism spectrum.

Let's say you bring in $2,000 after taxes each month, and your expenses are $1,500. Your goal is to save a total of $1,500 (your monthly expenses) x 9 months, which equals $13,500. Don't freak out over this number! It is a lot of money. But, when you eventually save it, you will feel so secure. Save nine months' worth of expenses, or any other number of months that makes sense to you. What is important is that you have money that you can rely on when – not if – you need it.

Where should you keep your emergency fund money? Put your monthly savings ($2,000 minus $1,500 equals $500 in our example) into a separate savings account if you are not charged fees at your bank or credit union. Or, put the money in a money market fund. Then be disciplined and do not raid your stash unless you are going through an emergency!

Do not keep the money at home. First, it is too easy to use the money for unimportant things when you have such easy access to it. A second reason to keep it in a financial institution is so you don't lose your hard-earned cash in the distressing event your home is broken into.

Allow your emergency fund to be your shield from worry. It is common to have an unexpected need for cash. Be prepared for that need.

I feel it is important to pay down debt *and* build an emergency fund at the same time. Not doing both simultaneously can cause you a future problem. Having debt and not saving for an emergency can financially sink you when you run into a problem. On the other hand, saving for an emergency and not paying off your debt will substantially add to your debt.

Please speak to your tax advisor if you have any questions.

What is a FICO score?

A few paragraphs ago, I wrote about FICO scores. What is a FICO score? It is your credit worthiness. Your score is determined by numerous factors, among them: paying your bills on time, including your credit cards; how much of your available credit, percent-wise, you are using; how long a credit history you have; and, etc.

FICO scores range from 300 - 850 points. Your number will determine whether you will receive a car or mortgage loan and the interest rate you will pay; whether the company where you interview for a job will hire you; how much you pay for car and home insurance; and, etc. The lower your score, the higher an interest rate you will pay on any loan you might secure and the more you will have to dish out for car and home insurance. An "excellent" number is between 730 and 850.

It is never too late to raise your FICO score.

The fourth step to financial independence is taking advantage of your company's retirement program.

If your company offers you a 401(k) plan, definitely participate in it. There are three large positives to a 401(k): first, the money you put into it will not be taxed immediately (but will be taxed when you take it out); second, your employer is giving you free money; and third, 401(k) money is a form of forced savings for your retirement.

The first point is self-explanatory.

Let's look at an example regarding the second point. Say your employer is matching 50 percent, up to the first six percent of your salary that you put into your 401(k) each year. In this example, you are earning $20,000 per year and you are putting in six percent of your salary into your 401(k), which is $1,200. Your company is then adding $600 to your 401(k) that year. The matching 50 percent, in this case $600, is the free money your employer is giving you. Why would you not want to take free money? If you cannot put in the full match, put in what you are able to. Then, when you receive a raise, let's say four percent, start putting half of your raise into your 401(k). Do not put more than the matched amount into this account. If you can afford to save extra money, open a regular IRA, a Roth IRA, or a non-IRA at a financial institution. You can choose the types of investments you want, rather than settling for the limited choices in your company's 401(k). If you have any questions, speak to your company's human resources department.

Every company has a "vesting" period. That means that if you voluntarily leave or are fired before that time – usually three or five years – you will not be able to keep the free money your company added to your 401(k), but you will, of course, keep the money you put into your own 401(k), plus or minus the amount your investments rose or fell. If you leave your job after you are fully vested, all of the free money and the amount of money you put in, plus or minus the amount your investments rose or fell, is yours.

Third point: When the money you invest into your 401(k) is automatically debited from your paycheck, you won't miss it. It is easy to spend money on "stuff." This forced savings will build over time, and you will be very happy to have those funds when you retire.

In my opinion, the easiest and best way to invest your money in your 401(k) is in an index mutual fund, which is known as passive investing. Over time, actively managed funds do not perform as well as passive index funds. I believe it's best to keep things simple.

If you work for a for-profit company like Citigroup, Verizon, IBM, etc., I recommend putting a maximum of five percent of your company's stock into your 401(k). When the stock eventually falls (stocks can rise and fall dramatically), you will appreciate having kept your money in different investment baskets. I have known of people who invested 50 percent of their 401(k) in their company's stock. When stocks took a huge hit in 2008-2009, some of these employees had losses they could not easily come back from.

Financial markets go up and down. Over time, if you want your money to do well, keep your 401(k) in index funds.

If you have any questions, a human resources representative from your company may be able to help you, or you can speak to your tax advisor.

When you no longer work for your company, **do not** cash out of your 401(k) or have the company write you a check. I have invested funds with both Fidelity Investments and Vanguard. You could contact either of them, or another investment company, and ask how to transfer your 401(k) funds into their plans. You can transfer the funds to either a regular IRA or a Roth IRA.

As mentioned earlier, you will not have to pay taxes on a regular IRA until after you take money out when you retire. With a Roth IRA, taxes are paid the tax year after you invest money into that account. Because you pay taxes when you put the money in, you will not have to pay taxes when you take the money out when you retire. Paying taxes on a Roth IRA can be a lot of upfront money, but you will have the benefit of not paying taxes on the money you take out of that account when you retire.

Before you transfer your retirement money to an investment company, you will have to fill out the investment company's forms. The money will then go directly into your new account at their institution. They will not manage the money for you; you will have to make the choices yourself. The positive aspect of transferring your 401(k) to them when you are no longer with your company is that you will have many more investment choices. Again, I recommend index funds, preferably spreading your money across a large-cap index fund, a mid-cap index fund, and a small-cap index fund. There are many books that can teach you how to choose an index fund. Many people try to invest their money in very complicated fashions. Do it simply and effectively. Index funds, in my opinion, are the way to go.

Please speak to your tax advisor before you move funds into a regular IRA or a Roth IRA.

To feel financially secure in your life, eliminate debt and build an emergency fund. And, to keep yourself from worry after you retire, contribute to your company's 401(k) while you have the opportunity.

Chapter 9

"Disconnection" and the Increasing Number of People on the Spectrum

Despite the best efforts of many on the autism spectrum, we fall short of our dreams.

Between high school and their early twenties, a large percentage of those on the spectrum are "disconnected," which means we are not continuing our education or employment.

The A.J. Drexel Autism Institute, Drexel University, put together the *National Autism Indicators Report: Transition into Young Adulthood*: 2015. In the first zero to two years after high school, 66 percent of those on the spectrum did not work or attend school; between two and four years after leaving high school, the number drops to 42 percent; at four to six years, the number is 23 percent; and, at six to 10 years, it's down to 3 percent.[8]

Those on the autism spectrum have quite a few challenges, which is why more of us are disconnected than those with other disabilities.

"Young adults on the Autism spectrum had far higher rates of disconnection than their peers with other disabilities. Less than 8% of young adults with a learning disability, emotional disturbance, or speech-language impairments were disconnected, compared to 37% of those with autism," said the A.J. Drexel Autism Institute's report.[9]

Furthermore, the National Autism Indicators Report said that between high school and our early twenties, 81% of those on the spectrum never lived independently.[10]

The report concludes with two disheartening thoughts, "We do not know why so many youth are not connecting to work and continued education after high school."[11] And, "Our knowledge base virtually ends at the age of 25."[12]

* * *

Every two years since the year 2000, the Centers for Disease Control and Prevention (CDC) has surveyed the number of eight-year-old children with autism spectrum disorder (ASD). In 2000, 1 in 150 children were on the spectrum in a six-state region.[13] The latest survey was conducted in 2020, and its results were disseminated in March 2023. Those figures estimate that 1 in 36 children now have ASD.[14] For every girl on the autism spectrum, 3.8 boys are also on the spectrum.[15]

In 2020, sites in 11 states were used for this study: Arizona, Arkansas, California, Georgia, Maryland, Minnesota, Missouri, New Jersey, Tennessee, Utah, and Wisconsin.[16]

Even with the increase in children with ASD, **the CDC is likely underestimating** the number of children with this disorder. In 2016, the CDC website said, "The CDC tracking system is likely not over-estimating the prevalence of ASD."[17] "…we are likely not counting some children with ASD."[18] Since the time this quote was published, the number of eight-year-old children with ASD has increased.

I believe that underestimating is still quite possible because there is such a wide disparity between the percentage of children found to have ASD across the 11 states in the study. Maryland had the largest percentage with 1 in 23.1 children per 1,000 children, while California had the lowest percentage with 1 in 44.9 children.[19]

In a very positive development, the CDC has begun tracking 16-year-olds. According to the study, "Follow-up of 16-year-olds is a new activity for the ADDM [Autism and Developmental Disabilities Monitoring] Network, and will help inform public health strategies to improve identification of, and services for, children with ASD. Tracking 16-year-old adolescents with ASD can also provide valuable information on transition planning in special education services and the planned trajectory for post-high school years."[20] This development began in 2018.

The CDC plans to publish the data in the near future. This information can be quite beneficial for those in, and completing, high school.

This new information should help lower the disconnection rate in the autism community.

For the first time, the CDC has estimated the number of people 18 years of age and older on the autism spectrum: 5,437,988 adults, or 2.21 percent of the United States population, are on the spectrum. Approximately 4,357,667, or 3.62 percent of men, and 1,080,322, or 0.86 percent of women have this disorder. This study was conducted in 2017 and published in May 2020.[21]

This information is quite important because, as the report states, "ASD is a lifelong condition, and many adults with ASD need ongoing services and support. The finding from this study can help states determine the need for diagnosing and providing services to adults in the United States who remain unidentified with ASD."[22]

This new information about the number of adults on the autism spectrum will assist those in need, giving them hope to keep their dreams alive and their lives rewarding.

What can society do to prevent human wasting? Perhaps have a set of supports in place after a student graduates from high school until they no longer need assistance. It may take decades for an autistic high school graduate to learn all the skills necessary to be successful in life. There is a lot to learn: grooming, how to find a job, communication at work and socially, keeping a home, budgeting, relationships, etc.

When a doctor does not diagnose a disease fully, their patient may not recover. People on the autism spectrum need appropriate support until they can maneuver through life without extensive help.

Chapter 10

Subtext/Be Smart/ We Are Not Robots

Many people believe we aren't intelligent because we have autism and lack street smarts. Yes, we may be book smart and have a large vocabulary, but "common sense" is often missing, my family would say.

When I was in my early teens, I was told numerous times by my mother and stepfather that I lacked common sense. That wasn't the problem. I didn't understand subtext, the real meaning behind words. My best example of this occurred in junior high school. One morning, I was late and missed the school bus. Jerry, my stepfather, was in a rush to go to work, but he agreed to take me to school.

"Take me the way the bus goes," he said. So I did. Right down a dead-end street. He screamed at me and was soooo mad. Who in their right mind would send someone down a dead-end street? I would.

The way I saw it was that I followed Jerry's directions, so why should he be upset? A portion of the bus driver's route was down a dead-end street, then the bus turned around. If Jerry would have said, "Take me to your school," I would have taken him straight to the school.

I was too literal then, but I have made progress. However, even now, because of autism, I still don't always understand subtext. I am in my early 60s. After all my life experiences, I hopefully won't make that kind of error again.

Yet mistakes happen to everyone. The best thing is to learn from them and move on.

If neurotypicals would speak to us in a more direct fashion, without subtext, that would definitely assist us and lead to far less confusion on everyone's part. Communication is a two-way street.

By the way, that story was Jerry's favorite to tell his friends. At his surprise 75th birthday party, I shared that dead-end adventure with a roomful of people. Of all the stories told that night, other attendees said it was the best tale.

* * *

Besides being unable to discern subtext, I have for most of my life trusted in others before they earned it.

Until recently, I trusted everyone until they gave me a reason not to. This is backwards from the way most of society behaves. For most people, trust is a slow process and must be earned.

If you let them (or don't know how to protect yourself), many people may take advantage of you. Only after an extended period will you know if you can really trust someone. Keep your secrets to yourself until you feel they will be safe with another person. Be smart about whom you share information with. I discuss this more in *Chapter 13: Don't Be a Sucker.*

* * *

Neurotypicals might be surprised to learn that those on the autism spectrum are not robots. What do I mean? Of course we are not robots, we are humans. But, many people not on the spectrum have expressed astonishment to discover that we have feelings and can be hurt emotionally. They are even further amazed that we have dreams and hopes and desires. We are more than what we seem to them.

Autistics want many of the same things that neurotypicals want, we just have difficulty expressing how we feel and what is in our hearts. Also, we don't use body language, which confuses those without autism.

We care about the world around us and have empathy for others. Why is this such a surprise to those not on the spectrum?

Perhaps because we live lives of routine. Personally, I eat the same cereals with water every morning. I go to the same restaurants and order the same food. I don't go out of my way to meet new people. At parties, I am very uptight, and if I am not sitting a good distance from others, I am at least mentally far away. I don't express joy and happiness, thus my feelings are often a mystery to others. Many of us with autism enjoy computers and machines because they are predictable. We are very direct, which can make us seem unfeeling.

Neurotypicals might do well to learn to dig deeper and discover who we really are. They could be surprised to know that we are actually quite similar to them.

Chapter 11

How to Develop Friendships

Loneliness and autism go hand-in-hand. Few of us have friends: a person to do things with, a confidant with whom to share our feelings, someone just to hang out with. Everyone else seems to be invited to parties, weddings, or a Saturday night out with the "guys" or "gals." Most of the time, we are alone in our room if we live with our parents, or by ourselves in our apartments or houses.

Since elementary school, I have been alone, except for brief periods when I socialized with groups in high school and college. When I was in sixth grade, a senior citizen who lived next door to me in my apartment building inquired, "Why don't you have any friends over?" I didn't want to tell her the reason, that I didn't have any friends.

Unfortunately, my lack of friendships has continued throughout my life. I have lived in the Phoenix area since 2005 and have only one person I hang out with once or twice a month. I am friendly with the staff at my banks and the library I visit. We say hello and sometimes talk a little. On occasion, I ask if they would like to go out for lunch or dinner. I always hear the same answer: "No."

I am not alone in my separation from others.

Going back to the *National Autism Indicators Report: Transition into Young Adulthood*: 2015, produced by the A.J. Drexel Autism Institute, Drexel University, "Approximately one in four young adults with autism were socially isolated. They never saw or talked with friends and were never invited to social activities within the past year."[23]

Why does this problem exist? Most likely because those on the autism spectrum lack awareness and understanding of social skills and body language. We act differently from neurotypicals: we don't look at the person we are speaking to, we are very literal because we have little understanding of subtext, and we don't recognize facial expressions, body language, and tone of voice.

With counseling and years of practice, we can improve our communications skills. Will it be enough knowledge to give us a boatful of friends? In my personal experience, no. But who needs a boat when a canoe will do? What I mean by that is that I have learned that if a person has one or two really good friends, they can feel extremely lucky.

What can we do to find more friends? One suggestion is to visit the "Meetup" website where persons with similar interests get together both online and in person. They may have hundreds or more groups in your area on virtually any imaginable topic, from photography to writing to losing weight. Rather than searching for just one group, find as many as you can that interest you. If you don't see one that piques your interest, consider starting your own group.

Besides Meetup, there might be an autism group in your city, and you might be able to make one or more friends with someone there. At the very least, you can discuss your issues with like-minded individuals. On the southeast side of Phoenix, there is an autism group that met monthly before Covid and occasionally had a guest speaker. There was also "social time" to talk with others. Since Covid, this group meets twice a month: once a month on Zoom and once a month in person.

Perhaps you might meet a friend at your place of worship, while you are taking a college class, or through your senior or community center.

I never understood how neurotypicals can make friends so easily. It seems to come so naturally to them. Decades ago, I went hiking with a group. Five of us were in a car, and all the others were laughing and chatting. After the event, I learned that those people had just met each other that day. I was astonished. It appeared to me that they had all been friends for a while.

Most friendships are not meant to stand the test of time. Very few actually do. If you have one or two close friends for decades or throughout your lifetime, you are a fortunate person.

We are meant to know people for different periods of time: some we know for a short period of time, others for a medium period, and still others for a longer period. With all friendships, we likely have lessons to learn. We may also need someone to support us and, likewise, have the opportunity to support them. When the reason they are in our life evaporates, the friendship ends. Don't be sad if you experience this. Life intended it to be that way. Be joyous and smile in your heart that you had their support and love for however long they shared it with you.

A woman prayed to the Universe for someone to help her buy a new car. Then I came into her life. I did the research, showed her how she could afford to purchase the vehicle, and held her hand throughout the entire process, including negotiating with the sales manager when I was by her side.

Five days after she bought the car, we separated for six weeks. I came back into her life only to discover that she was planning on moving to the other side of the United States. I was happy that I could reunite with her peacefully and with love. We were, however, never meant to be long-term friends. I was grateful that she reopened areas of my heart and acted as my muse for a portion of this book. She was grateful that I was with her throughout the process of buying her car.

Allow yourself to let go of a friend if it's time for that friendship to end. Don't try to make it more than what it is. If this person is meant to be a forever-friend, it will happen.

What's the best way to make a friend and break out of the No-Friends box?

First, share who you are, but go very light with the personal information at the beginning. If you open up too quickly, the other person might be uncomfortable because they will feel obligated to share a great deal about themselves with you.

Second, learn to "chitchat." I define chitchat as unimportant conversation that fills up time, such as talking about the weather or a recent movie. Autistics rarely participate in chitchat. We have very narrow interests, for example, astronomy, dinosaurs, trains, etc. My expertise is in investments, national and international politics, and the world economy. I can talk for hours and hours about my favorite topics. After listening to us ramble for just a few minutes, a person not on the autism spectrum usually will have their fill and walk away or tune out.

Rather than talk endlessly about our favorite topics, we must expand our conversation into the dreaded chitchat. This kind of conversation builds trust and rapport with a neurotypical. Chitchatting is difficult for us because we generally don't talk to bond; our goal is to communicate in order to share information.

Third, improve your listening skills. No one wants to spend much time with a person who talks only about themselves or their interests. Being a friend is a two-way street. We must listen to the other person just like we want them to listen to us. Besides, no one knows everything. They might provide an interesting or very important piece of information.

You must not hog the conversation. Years ago, I visited a friend after work. He talked about his issues without taking a breath and not letting me get a word in. After 90 minutes, I got up to leave because I was tired of hearing about his negative life. He was surprised that I wanted to go. He then asked what was going on with me. But it was too late; I already decided to leave.

Fourth, combine your chitchatting with listening skills by asking questions of the other person. Have they seen any good movies lately? What kind of art do they like? Would they like to eat at your favorite Italian restaurant? Or, if they say they just arrived home from traveling, ask about their favorite destination.

Fifth, take a real interest in their passion. If they get excited about art, for example, ask to go with them when they attend an art fair or art museum. You may even check a book out from the library to learn more about their interest or research it on the internet.

Sixth, go out on your own to a park, shopping, zoo or anywhere else you enjoy going. It is often easier to meet someone when you are having fun doing something you enjoy because there is less stress, and you are being "natural." And if you don't meet anyone, that's OK, as long as you are having fun doing your own thing.

There are many opportunities to find friends if you stretch beyond your comfort zone. You will not find a new friend while you are sitting in your room or house hoping someone will come knocking on your door looking for you. (Waiting at home hasn't been a successful friend-making strategy for me – at least not yet!)

Try these tips. You will have a better chance of developing a friendship than if you keep doing what has not worked in the past. You have a lot to share with others. Go for it.

Chapter 12

The Positive Side

In the last few chapters, I have focused on the negative side of having autism. There are many positive aspects that are sometimes overlooked.

Being detailed is very helpful both in and out of the workplace. Making sure a job is done right no matter how detailed or repetitive, the person with autism can do it.

Years ago, when I was working as an editor, one of my responsibilities was to find errors in my own articles and other people's work. In my career, I made two mistakes in my newspaper articles that got past me. Not only did I edit well, I relished finding errors. I was almost gleeful about it.

Hand-in-hand with being detailed is having the ability to **focus on a task for hours** at a time. Before the Covid pandemic, I would drive to my local library nearly seven days a week to use the internet to check my e-mail and keep up with the news and my investments. I, like others with autism, can hyperfocus on a task for many hours. It is not unusual for me to work on my investments for four or five hours straight without moving. I am very much into my own world and do not notice the passage of time.

Both these last two points are also positives on the home front. Everything from toiling on finances for hours to remembering the type of flowers your partner likes will be appreciated.

Resistance to change is both positive and negative. On the positive side, a person with autism will stay at a company for years and accumulate a wide, deep, and detailed knowledge base. We can recall information that everyone else has long forgotten.

What is often extremely bothersome for those on the autism spectrum is change, until we get used to it. Learning computer software while I was working or volunteering always frustrated me until I was comfortable with the change. Then I was happy – until the IT department changed the software again. Actually, new computer software is one of two things that causes me to have a meltdown; the other is fragrance and chemical smells, such as new carpet. When I encounter these, I become uncontrollably upset. Beyond computers, for years I was very, very uncomfortable with any changes in my routine. Now that I am older, I deal better with change. I am not always as flexible as others want me to be, but better than when I was younger.

Perhaps because autistics don't like change, we are very *loyal*. We often will stay at a job for many years, which has obvious benefits for employers and for us. We don't go looking for "greener pastures" and are very happy to stay with our company. This loyalty also extends to our mates. Personally, I have never cheated on a girlfriend, even when an opportunity presented itself. I am not aware of having met any autistic person who wasn't loyal to their partner, although, of course, it could happen.

Honesty is another attribute that those on the autism spectrum possess. We are honest to our core, sometimes too honest for neurotypicals. If you want a "real" answer to your question, ask someone with autism. Problems can occur because most neurotypicals do not want an honest answer. We are missing the "white lie" filter.

Those on the autism spectrum see the world much more in black and white and much less in gray, or the middle ground, than neurotypicals. Either the person we are acquainted with is honest or they or not. "Little white lies" are disastrous for any kind of relationship with us because they break the bonds of trust. "If Suzi is lying to me now, how do I know she won't lie about other things," we think.

When my sister and I were young, our father wanted to take us for a second canoe trip on the Current River in southern Missouri. Before we went on the trip, my mother told us she was very much against us going canoeing because she feared there would be an accident and we would drown. My father tried to get us to go and tell our mother a white lie by saying we'd only gone camping. I couldn't lie to my mother. My father was disappointed that we didn't spend time on the river.

Lastly, we are not like the general population because ***we are always our true selves***. When I am in a relationship, after the fifth month or so, I see major personality shifts with the person I am dating that were not immediately apparent. I think, "Who is this person?" Neurotypicals feel comfortable after a period of time, so they "let their guard down." People on the autism spectrum are consistently more real. I tell those I meet, "Who you see now is the same person I will be later." Being one's true self is more honest and less confusing to your partner. In my experience, most neurotypicals do not feel this way.

Chapter 13

Sugarcoated

Neurotypicals often try to sugarcoat negative information. I think they feel that doing so will soften undesirable communication. I believe that in conversations between neurotypicals, this indirect approach often works. After all, why suffer the sharpness of a sword when a pinprick will do?

As mentioned previously, indirectness to a person on the autism spectrum is the same as lying because it shades the truth. And anything that makes reality more difficult to comprehend is an impediment to understanding for an autistic person.

A "friend" sugarcoated information when she told me that we would not be "an item." However, she said, there was a chance we could be a couple in the future. To make sure I heard her correctly, I asked her a detailed question, which she answered affirmatively. I thought, "OK, maybe with time and a bit of luck we could merge our lives together." The next day, she revealed to me that she had "sugarcoated" her words. In reality, I had virtually no measurable opportunity for a relationship with her. She said that she could not tell me why, but then she spoke about my health. I felt that her so-called kindness to me was far worse than if she would have just been honest in the first place. I felt she had misled me on purpose. On our first date, I told her I do not understand subtext, the hidden but real meaning behind words. I need directness. I think she knew that honesty would hurt me and wanted to spare my feelings.

Do not sugarcoat your words with someone with autism. We will trust you if you are honest with us, even if you tell us what we don't want to hear. At least we will not feel we were led to believe a falsehood if you are straight with your words, no matter how unhappy we may feel about what you are saying.

When I presented a neurotypical acquaintance with the above situation, she explained, "It's not about being truthful; it's about being brutally honest. People say things without trying to be mean; rather, they are attempting to spare feelings. If you don't pick up on those nuances, you think people are lying, when it's actually just a method of communication most people engage in."

Perhaps this is why neurotypicals think we are blunt and rude in our communication? They are subtle. We are the bull in a china shop. They avoid the truth so they don't hurt the other person. We always tell the truth in order to be honest. These two communication styles usually don't mix-and-match.

What is the solution? Perhaps both sides can try to meet somewhere in the middle. Perhaps neurotypicals can be more forthright, and we can be more subtle. If they can avoid white lies, we won't feel misled. Communication is all about coming together to be understood.

Chapter 14

Faulty Connections

A "we" relationship is physically and spiritually higher than a one-way connection where the focus of the relationship is solely on one person's needs, as opposed to both partners helping each other reach their physical and spiritual goals. Relationships are a "we," while a one-way connection is an "I".

My Uncle Sidney began a program that fed lunch to needy seniors five days a week. He also worked on many other projects for seniors. During my Aunt Annie's eulogy, the religious leader said that my Uncle Sidney could not have participated in these activities and numerous other social programs without her support. They propped each other up and encouraged growth.

At the time of this writing, I am 63 years old. I have been in a variety of "I" connections, from as brief as six-and-a-half weeks to seven years. Most of these centered on me trying to please my partner while they often ignored my happiness and growth.

Please don't misunderstand me. It is wonderful to focus on the other person, to make them happier and uplift them. I feel joyous when I can make my partner's life easier and happier.

My problem is that I would almost idolize them and put their needs far above my own. With one woman, for example, I helped her with almost everything in her life: her college studies, making everyday household decisions, and investing her retirement funds for her. The most painful and challenging hurdle we faced together was when we found out she had cancer. I was just about to break up with her when we learned about her diagnosis and that she would need an operation. Instead of leaving, I stayed with her through her procedure and six months of chemo. Those were traumatic times for both of us. When she was in remission, had found a job, and was physically stable again, she gave me a difficult time one night because I was unable to go bicycle riding with her because of my asthma. I wasn't very healthy, according to her. We broke up that night.

Those on the autism spectrum are particularly susceptible to being taken advantage of, most likely because we are honest and naturally want to help others. Because we are that way, we believe others are honest and want to help us, too. A few neurotypicals have those positive qualities. In my experience though, an unfortunate number do not.

Years before my girlfriend had cancer, I was in a car accident on a Saturday afternoon on an interstate. After the ambulance transported me to a hospital, I called my girlfriend and asked her to come to the hospital to be with me. She said "no" because she had plans to celebrate one of my ex-girlfriends' birthdays at a restaurant.

I put up with that kind of selfishness for quite a while with several women in my life. They were interested in what they needed. If their wants correlated with what I wanted, we both had our needs met. Rarely would any of them do something I needed that they did not want to do. They also infrequently helped me reach my physical and spiritual dreams, the whole point of a "we" relationship.

Relationships are about give-and-take. I have always dated women who would take, but could not, or would not, give in return.

Heather Olsen, my friend who is an energy healer with psychic and medium abilities, recently taught me that I am important and worthy of a healthy relationship. Even though I was mentally aware of these concepts, I did not believe in them, perhaps because of all of the negativity showered upon me for the majority of my life.

If you do not treat yourself with caring and respect, others will not treat you with caring and respect.

I am trying to think of an example of when I had a "we" relationship. While I have had numerous "I" connections, I find it instructive that I do not have an example of a personal "we" relationship. Now that I have worked on my internal self, I believe I am ready for a new, healthy type of connection.

Everyone should look for a person who will help them grow physically and spiritually, have happiness blossom, and be able to compromise with them.

Search for and pursue "we" relationships. Let the "I" connections pass you by. You are worth much more than those.

Chapter 15

Eliminate Sadness

If anything will inhibit a person's progress in this world, it is sadness. As autistic persons, we are fighting loneliness, being misunderstood, and being bullied. Everywhere we turn, we find problems and miscommunications, both small and large.

Sadness is common for those with autism because we are alone in life, even when we do not want to be. It is uncommon for us to have a multitude of friends. Being alone in this world often causes sadness. Some of us are lucky to have more than one friend we can call on the phone or hang out with. Some autistics have no friends. Personally, my number of friends is very small. I spend time with the same person approximately once or twice a month and feel fortunate we are connected.

Please read *Chapter 11: How to Develop Friendships* when you are feeling lonely. That section can hopefully guide you to finding one or more friends, which can bring you happiness.

It is time to step out of your sadness box.

It has been a few years since sadness began to lift from my being. No, mood-enhancing drugs (prescriptions, if you prefer) are not what solved the problem. Although drugs did elevate me in my darkest times, they did not eliminate my sadness.

Once again, I have Heather Olsen to thank for pulling me out of my sadness. When I gave her credit for this, she texted, "All I did was believe in you and teach you how to believe in yourself." Maybe it was that simple, maybe not. I don't know.

The first step in tearing away the darkness, Heather taught me, is believing everyone has worth. Why do we have worth? Simply because we exist. It took thought and effort by both G-d and then our parents to create us. G-d created us out of love. And, if we are fortunate, our parents did also.

A step beyond that thought: We are important to this world and in G-d's eyes. Like most others, we are a positive force in this world.

G-d did not put us on Earth to be sad. Yes, bad things happen to all of us, and most of us temporarily get blue and discouraged when negative events occur. If we are the "normal" level of happy, or at least not excessively sad or depressed, we will bounce back to our regular selves following a challenging event.

Beauty is a source of happiness. One source of beauty is art, including painting. Not everyone can paint like the masters. I have always wanted to be able to paint well. What I visualize in my mind is far different than what I can express on canvas. A few lucky souls are fantastic painters. Their work brings joy and wonder into this world and into our lives. Without this type of beauty, the world would be a little less complete.

Everyone has a reason for being here on Earth. We may not know what our reason is yet, but over time we might determine our purpose in life. Meditation helps us still our minds so we can find the answers we seek.

Challenges occur in our lives so we can learn the lesson(s) we came here for. Have you noticed that unless we learn how to solve a problem (i.e., not make the same mistake again and again), that the situation keeps recurring throughout our lives?

As I wrote in the last chapter, one of my challenges is romantic relationships. I connect with those who think about the "I" in the connection, rather than the "we." I have done this all my life. I never knew how to stand up for myself until recently. If we believe, truly believe, that we are worthy of a positive, loving mate, we will have a better chance of connecting with one.

Every person sends vibrations into the universe and attracts what they deep down believe they deserve. If you don't like what is coming to you, you need to change your beliefs. Your thoughts will follow your new beliefs, and then attraction will occur. Don't just give it lip service. Take steps to actively change your beliefs.

There are ways to improve your beliefs about yourself. First, communicate with people who are spiritually higher. They can help you see a different path than the one you are now traveling. Spiritually advanced people, or stepping stones, as I like to call them, will come into your life when you are ready to make a change. You might meet them at your place of worship, a volunteer organization, school, or yoga practice. One of my doctors knew I needed spiritual help, so he guided me to Heather.

Second, meditate. Answers can come out of stillness and calm. Meditate once or twice a day for approximately 10 minutes each time. The idea is to stop thinking and just be in stillness. There are many, many ways to meditate. First, turn off your cellphone, be in a quiet environment, and limit all distractions. Second, sit in a relaxed position. Third, close your eyes and think of nothing. When a thought enters, gently sweep it away until you are thinking of nothing again.

It may take a while to learn to allow yourself to relax enough to meditate. No one can say exactly how long it will take to begin working for you. Practice going within yourself, away from the noise and speed of your surroundings. We have all the answers within ourselves to the questions that are most important to us.

Let's talk about breathing, both while meditating and not meditating. Most people's breath is too shallow because they breathe in only down to their chest. The better way to breathe is through your diaphragm. This also takes practice. Start by paying attention to your breathing.

* * *

Being isolated from others will often magnify sadness. Spend time with family or friends. If you can't be with them physically, talk with them on a cellphone or write to them on a computer. These types of communication can make you feel better.

Focusing on doing something nice for someone you know or helping a stranger can also help alleviate sadness.

Nine years ago, I was told I have cancer, so I began taking infusions. A Phoenix organization called The Joy Bus delivered a meal to me once a week that was cooked by a chef. The paper bag that held the food had words and/or pictures written and/or drawn by an elementary school student. To get my dreary focus off myself, I wrote a thank you letter to the student who wrote encouraging words on one of my paper bags. I felt better after writing the letter. I hope the letter also made her feel good.

Volunteering is also a wonderful way to help others and change our focus from ourselves. When we are thinking of others, we deflect sadness, and our mood will be elevated.

There are numerous opportunities to volunteer in most communities. A personal favorite of mine is food banks. Because I have gone without food for extended periods of time, once as a student at the University of Missouri-Columbia, and a second time shortly after I completed college, I find it important to help others facing the same challenge.

Nearly every nonprofit needs help. Do you enjoy being with children? There are many agencies you can volunteer with. Animals? What about seniors? Ill patients in a hospital or a nursing home? Cancer organizations need assistance. The list is almost endless.

Even a small gesture may be seen as something major by the recipient of our good deeds. None of us fully understands how our presence affects others. Goodness spreads like water. Reading a book to an ill person in a hospital, talking to a scared child, petting an injured animal at an animal clinic, or serving food at a soup kitchen has enormous benefits. **Only you can share your gifts.**

I find that everything happens positively in the end, even when we believe we are having a bad experience. In 2022, I needed to have cancer infusions in October and November. The cost was high for me, more than $2,800 after insurance paid its portion of the bill. The company that did the infusions found two medical grants for me in 2023, but they covered future treatments, not the ones I took in 2022. I was quite concerned about the cost. Fortunately, I applied to the PAN Foundation. The grant was closed at the time, but one week later it opened, and the foundation covered my costly 2022 cancer infusions expenses.

Sadness is a problem not just for those with autism. It can, and does, afflict the general population. These solutions work the same way for everyone.

For those who are currently suicidal, please see your medical doctor, psychiatrist, and/or a therapist (please read *Chapter 21: It's Time to See a Therapist*). The therapist can use talk therapy, while the medical doctor and psychiatrist can suggest a prescription(s) which will remove the darker veils that are blocking positive light from reaching you. You will feel better. Once you do, you can move even further toward your dreams and goals. Your perspective will be different, and you will begin to appreciate all the wonderful things around you.

Chapter 16

Live a Balanced Life

There's a spiritual saying, "In one pocket, write a note, 'the world was made for me' and in the other pocket write, 'I am but dust and ashes.'"

Look at "the world was made for me" note when you are feeling insufficient. Do not visualize yourself as small or less important than anyone else. **This world was made for you.**

It is not correct to say, I am *only* doing (think of something you believe is insignificant) so-and-so, thus my contribution is much smaller than another person's. Your piece of the mosaic would be a hole if you weren't there to fill it. You cannot be replaced by anyone else.

Please learn to accept yourself. You are important!!!

This is not to say you cannot improve; of course you can. There is no area in life that cannot be made better, be it your workplace or your personal life. We can all be more thoughtful and considerate, listen more, try harder, be less stubborn. Although no one expects perfection, everyone does expect you to try your best. In areas where you feel you are deficient, or not as good as you'd like to be, focus on reaching your goal.

It has taken me many years to accept myself and be comfortable with who I am. It was not an easy task. I have had numerous challenges in my life: my childhood, growing up in a divorced family, constant bullying in junior high school, social difficulties, physical barriers, and autism. At times, it has felt like I have had too much to face. Even so, G-d doesn't give us more than we can handle. My solace is that all of these challenges have formed me into the person I am: unique and caring and insightful. I would never have become who I am today if I did not have the totality of my experiences, both good and bad.

Please look at the "I am but dust and ashes" note when you are too puffed up. Everyone, not just you, contains sparks of Holiness from the Infinite, though we sometimes forget this. Others' thoughts and opinions are just as important as yours, because everyone originates from Source. You are but one star out of billions.

You were born to learn certain lessons. Don't think of the lessons as big or small, important or trivial. As far as the Universe is concerned, lessons are all integral and equal.

It is best to live a balanced life, both in how you think of yourself in the world and how you act. Stay in the middle of the path.

Celebrate who you are. Go out into the world and be proud. Remember, though, that your contribution to this world is only one piece of a larger mosaic.

Balance your life and step out of your box.

Chapter 17

Autism and Sensitivity

Those on the autism spectrum can be very sensitive to sound, light, touch, and smells. I wrote this chapter to explain to those not on the spectrum what is going on in an autistic's mind. This will give you some understanding about how we are feeling and why we react to what neurotypicals often think is a normal situation.

This may seem unusual to some, but loud sounds are shattering for many of us on the spectrum, including myself. These sensitivities are not in our imagination, or preferences; they are real problems that cause pain and/or anxiety.

I can deal with crowd noise at a mall or baseball game. However, when I am in my local library 30 minutes, 15 minutes, and five minutes before it closes, there is a very, very loud message on a loudspeaker. I put my hands over my ears and wait for the announcement to finish. The stimuli is too forceful, and I get overwhelmed. The pain in my ears is jarring. Besides putting my hands over my ears when I hear the loudspeaker in the library, I also take deep breaths. That helps me calm down when I feel overloaded by the loud volume. This went on for some time, until eventually, I spoke with the library manager and asked her to lower the sound. Thoughtfully, she did. Lowering the sound helped calm me down.

Also at the library, I find it very distracting when people are talking. For years after I graduated from the University of Missouri-Columbia, it was rare for a library not to be silent. Unfortunately, libraries are becoming like most other public places: loud. Trying to concentrate on my work is difficult when crosscurrents of noise collects in my brain.

Maybe noise at an event does not bother me mentally because I am not trying to focus on my work.

Once while I was in a Hallmark store, I was unable to concentrate while I tried to read greeting cards because of the overwhelmingly loud music streaming out of the loudspeakers. The thoughts on paper were not complicated, they were only greeting cards. I asked one of the employees if the music could be turned off because it was making me unable to concentrate. I also shared with her that I have autism.

After she spoke with her manager, the concert-like volume was turned off for only five minutes, but it was enough time for me to find the perfect cards.

The effect of the loud music on me in this instance was that I couldn't understand what the sentences on the greeting cards meant. Yes, it was weird. But in the end, I was able to read the cards, locate the best ones, buy them, and hopefully bring joy to the recipients. Everyone won because I spoke up and the manager made an exception for me.

My mother has a ceiling fan in her den, which is directly below the bedroom I used to live in. The whirring sound was so loud when the fan was on that I could not sleep. If I turned it off when I went to bed and then someone turned it on in the morning, the hum of the whirling fan blades would immediately wake me up, even though no one in the den could hear the sound. After hearing me ask incessantly, my mother and stepfather eventually agreed not to turn on the fan while I was asleep.

Fluorescent lights are another irritant, as they have a strange buzzing noise that bothers many people with autism.

One of my acquaintances, who is also on the autism spectrum, has a terrible time with the fluorescent light itself, not just the sound emanating from the bulbs. She described the flickering of the lights as similar to a disco ball.

Other autistics hate the feel of certain fabrics on their skin. I have heard of some people on the spectrum taking off all their clothes as soon as they arrive home just to alleviate the irritation of the clothing against their skin.

Touch also includes unwanted hugs. One of my relatives always hits my back several times with her hands when she hugs me. It hurts. Others want to hug me way too tightly, which also causes pain. If I want a hug, I will let you know.

Some of us enjoy hugs, some don't. It is always best to ask.

When Covid began, I altered my routine to stay home four or five days a week. On the internet, I have read that many people had a very difficult time staying isolated because they were without physical connection with friends and family. Most autistics, including myself, are much happier to have less contact with others. Being around most people is aggravating, although sometimes we wish to have people around.

Chemical smells cause me to have a meltdown. Odors like fragrances, cigarette smoke, cleaning compounds, and new carpet drive me to distraction. Don't even try to put me in a room with a brand new or recently cleaned carpet. It generally takes one year before the carpet odor dissipates enough for me to find it tolerable.

The only way I am aware of dealing with my sensitivity is to ask for help like I did at the library and the Hallmark store. Many times, those not on the spectrum will work with us, although sometimes they will not be able to or want to. If people are unwilling to make the situation better for me, I walk away.

Chapter 18

Autism and OCD

Not only can a person be on the autism spectrum, but they may also struggle with an added condition(s), as well. These additional condition(s) are called comorbidities.

This second obstacle may take a number of forms: Obsessive Compulsive Disorder (OCD), depression, Attention Deficit Hyperactivity Disorder (ADHD), anxiety, etc.

According to DSM-5, "Many individuals with autism spectrum disorder have psychiatric symptoms that do not form part of the diagnostic criteria for the disorder (about 70% of individuals with autism spectrum disorder may have one comorbid mental disorder, and 40% may have two or more comorbid mental disorders)."[24]

It is not uncommon for a person with autism also to have OCD. In an article in **SpectrumNews.org**, Per Hove Thomsen, clinical professor of psychiatry, at the Psychiatric Hospital for Children and Adolescents at Aarhus University in Denmark, "reported that up to 17 percent of Danish children with OCD display mild symptoms of autism."[25]

What are the symptoms of OCD? Having the same thoughts enter your mind again and again. A second part of OCD that a person may or may not experience involves counting and/or touching. An example is making sure the front door is locked. The person with OCD will not check it once or twice; they may verify that the door is locked 10 times, 100 times, or more.

A second example is washing one's hands to kill any possible germs. The ritual is not finished until the person with OCD feels internally comfortable. These rituals are necessitated by the belief that "something bad" will occur if the ritual is not completed. Completing the ritual eases anxiety.

For a person with OCD, reading may also involve the ritual of counting. For instance, performing mental gymnastics with the periods or commas on a page, or applying a numerical value to various letters in a sentence. This particular ritual was devastating to me while I was in college. I love books and the knowledge contained within the pages. I wanted desperately to read and learn but couldn't because my OCD rituals held me back. It affected the length of time it would take me to read a page and understand what I was reading and caused me to read much more slowly than my professors expected. In my sophomore year, I was reading only about 25 to 30 pages per class each semester, which is a ridiculously low number. I should have been reading and taking notes on thousands of pages on each subject. Although OCD was a major part of my life, I still somehow managed to complete the requirements for a bachelor's degree and an additional year of graduate work.

Very unfortunately, OCD still affects my reading, and even the writing of this book. My counselor does not understand why my rituals are worse for me with a physical book than reading on the computer.

I learn about the world through reading. I know far less than I would if I weren't affected by OCD, and I am sure I would have had a more solid career if I had completed my master's and Ph.D. degrees.

Hoarding is an additional problem that some with OCD experience. One of my friends drives long distances every weekend to buy several different newspapers. He doesn't read the newspapers – he just saves them. He has several stacks of newspapers that are almost my height, 6 feet.

If you know someone with OCD, do not interrupt them while performing a ritual because it will only multiply their anxiety and may force them to repeat the ritual from the beginning. The more stress I feel, the more rituals I need to do. Unfortunately, they are not like chores. Completing a ritual does not mean it is finished for the day. Obsessions and rituals continue throughout the majority of a person's waking hours.

When I was younger, I was considered "different," "weird," and "strange" because I did not have the ability to communicate well because I am autistic. OCD added a layer of bizarreness to my behavior and contributed to my social isolation.

OCD can be quite destructive. Reducing rituals will greatly increase a person's quality of life. When I was in my twenties, I felt like I was wasting my life. Each ritual can take a long time. Sadly, there were multiple daily rituals which squandered the majority of my days.

I know of two ways to diminish the effects of OCD: medication and Cognitive Behavioral Therapy (CBT).

In my mid-forties, I began taking two prescriptions to reduce anxiety. The medications diminished my constant nervousness, so my need to perform rituals were dramatically reduced. An additional benefit was that I was able to fly on an airplane to visit my family. If you have OCD, you may want to speak to a psychiatrist to see if medication may be a solution for you.

The second possible way to reduce or eliminate OCD is Cognitive Behavioral Therapy. A therapist can talk to you about how you can alter your thoughts and behaviors to change your reality. The goal is to change your patterns. You can find a great deal of information about this topic on the internet or speak to your therapist to learn more.

Chapter 19

Stuck in the Past

Has your mind ever been stuck in a mental circle, going 'round and 'round about your past? It could be about your childhood, an ex-partner(s) who treated you badly, or how you wish you would have spent more time with your grandparents before they died. There are many opportunities to wander into memories.

If you daydream several times a day about events that previously happened to you, upset you, or you wish you could change, welcome to my previous world. I have finally been able to escape from my past.

The problem with constantly dwelling on what is behind you, as opposed to living in the present, is the stickiness of "what ifs." My life would have been drastically different IF I'd have asked her out on a date. What would have happened IF I'd had friends in elementary school? Everything would be different now IF I could have exchanged my sad life for a much more positive one.

It is difficult to get out of the glue of what if's and into the present. My Uncle Bob, a joke writer for Bob Hope and Phyllis Diller, wrote a note decades ago he posted in his business: "Diet is a four-letter word." My modern-day response is the word "past" is another four-letter word. Many people fight to move forward, to get past the past.

How can we walk through the door leading to the present?

First, forgive yourself for the mistakes you made. It is easy to look back and say, "I should have done this," or "I should have done that." Now that you are older and wiser, of course you would bypass the obstacle in the road that tripped you up in an earlier time. Fixing problems is effortless in hindsight. If you could do the right thing every time, from your birth until the present, you would remain static, because you would not need to improve. More to the point, there would have been no reason for you to be born. Mistakes give you the opportunity to make a better choice in the future when a similar situation arises. **Mistakes are how we grow.**

Second, meditate. Meditation will teach you how to focus on the here-and-now. Please read *Chapter 15: Eliminate Sadness* for information about how to meditate and breathe properly.

You don't want to discover, while examining your past, that you have been paralyzed for 30 years and have completed few or none of your dreams and goals. Live in and focus on the present. Then, near the end of your life, when you think about your happy memories, they will be much sweeter.

Chapter 20

Autism and Depression

Are you sad most of the time and feeling as though you are just taking up space on this planet? Do you have thoughts about wanting to end your life? Depression is a serious condition that at the very least limits your positivity and, at worst, is a negative force that can cause you to kill yourself.

I believe having autism makes you more susceptible to depression. Why? Because autistics are for the most part socially isolated. I am not a medical doctor or a social worker, but it appears that the effects of autism and poor communication skills lead to very few friends, or none at all, which in turn causes sadness and then depression.

According to DSM-5, "Adolescents and adults with autism spectrum disorder are prone to anxiety and depression."[26]

I have not been able to find statistics about how many people with autism commit suicide. However, I did locate a rare study in a medical journal about autism, depression, and suicidal thoughts.

Data was collected from a specialist diagnostic clinic in England from Jan. 23, 2004 through July 8, 2013. In the study, 374 adults (256 men and 118 women) had autism. Two hundred forty-three of 367 (66 percent) self-reported suicidal ideation; 127 of 365 (35 percent) self-reported plans or attempts at suicide; and 116 of 368 (31 percent) self-reported depression.[27]

It seems odd at first glance that fewer people admitted being depressed than having thoughts, plans, or attempts at suicide. The depression number could be lower than the suicidal ideation and plans, or suicide attempts, because those on the autism spectrum have a difficult time explaining to others how they feel.

The study authors also noted, "Adults with Asperger's syndrome were significantly more likely to report lifetime experience of suicidal ideation than were individuals from a general UK population sample, people with one, two, or more medical illnesses, or people with psychotic illness."[28]

Why are these percentages much higher than the general population? I am convinced it is not only because we are socially isolated, but most of us are unemployed, and a large number of us lack self-esteem.

Sadness blocks out hope, which in the long run leads to despair and depression. If you are depressed, you will choose not to follow your natural trail of movement, exploration, and joy.

It is easy to follow a negative mental path and curl up in your bed expecting the rain never to end. Rather than following that path, focus on what you are grateful for and what you enjoy doing. What brings you contentment? Playing with cats? Cooking? Walking in a forest?

If you perceive your life as having the potential of good things around the corner, your attitude will be positive. You will choose better paths to follow, thus making the potential for happiness far more likely.

Allow me to share an example with you. You have cancer and your doctor recommends chemo. If you perceive the chemo as a gift from the Universe, you will have a more positive attitude. You will talk more to your friends about the process, you will eat more, and you will know you have a good chance of beating your cancer. If you perceive the chemo as poison, your mind and body will limit your chances of healing. (I have personal experience with cancer, not chemo.)

Often, looking outside yourself will help get you out of your rut. Take your dog or cat to a senior center or a foster care community and let the residents pet and play with your animal. Volunteer to cook at a homeless shelter. Paint and donate your artwork to an organization having a silent auction so the money can be used to support your favorite cause. You will feel good about helping others.

Any kind of exercise will also help you shed the depression, from walking to swimming to running. Just get up and move.

Too many autistics are depressed, and many think about suicide.

If you can begin to perceive the world in a more positive way, over time your outlook will improve. I am not saying that you will get everything, or even most of what you want, but your life will be happier. The more positive you are, the more positivity you will attract. Negative events happen to everyone; that is how life works. Changing your perception of those events will alter your attitude and can convert a rocky path to a smoother one.

If you stay emotionally closed, no one will appreciate you. If you open up, your joy will spread far beyond what you might ever expect.

I had been sad and depressed for most of my life. My friend Heather and my Phoenix counselor helped to change my negative thoughts to much more positive ones. I also thank G-d for keeping me alive and allowing me to help others. If you remain optimistic, your life will be happier.

If you are too depressed for too long (both you and others around you will know when that is), get help from your medical doctor, psychiatrist, and/or therapist. Prescriptions and talk therapy can help you in the short and long run. Lots of people want to help you. Do not choose to fight your depression alone.

It's time to break out of your depression box.

Chapter 21

It's Time to See a Therapist

Sometimes life becomes too much: too much pain, too much aggravation, too much uncertainty. Sometimes you need help to navigate your journey.

There is no reason to walk through the forest alone, especially when assistance is available. When you fall, isn't it easier to get back up when someone is there to give you a hand? Of course it is. To follow this thought a little further, say you are with a guide in the forest when you see two paths. The guide has traveled both paths, so he knows what to expect if you follow either one. Why should you guess which way to go when your guide has experience not with one path, but with both?

A therapist can assist you when you are having a problem. His/her outstretched hand can help you avoid making a mistake (falling), understanding why you fell in the first place (insight), and talking about things to do so you don't fall again (avoid falling – or at least falling into that particular hole).

To continue just a bit further with this forest analogy, your chosen therapist can talk with you about your choices in a particular situation (paths you may not see well), point out the positives and negatives, and discuss the possible outcomes of your choices.

Therapists can help guide you through the Forest of Life. Do not feel embarrassed if you need help. At times, we all need help.

I first saw a therapist for four years beginning in third grade because my elementary school teacher recommended it. I began again my freshman year of college when I was overwhelmed with college life. I stopped for a few years until I moved back to St. Louis and continued again in the Phoenix area from 2005 to 2019.

My therapist told me I have come a long way in communication and my thought processes since I have been in Arizona. Others who have known me for decades have shared with me that I am communicating in a much clearer fashion now than I did 20 years ago.

I believe I am unusual for seeing a therapist for so long, but I have had multiple problems I wanted to unravel. I am finished with my therapy journey for now and am walking in the forest on my own.

Because I have so much experience working with therapists, I would like to suggest a few ways to find a "good match."

1. I have always contacted my health insurance company to see who is covered in my area. Then I look up the therapists online and see what others say about them.
2. What is the therapist's specialization? Children? Adults? Autism? Relationships? Does their skill set match up with your needs?
3. Do you open up better with a male or female?
4. What is your communication style? Do you want a therapist to ask you questions and speak infrequently, or would you rather they share their opinions with you?

After the first session, you should have some idea about whether you and your therapist are a good match. After the second session, you should definitely know. Do you feel comfortable with the person? Is the vibe right? Does their communication style work for you?

Do not be embarrassed if your first therapy relationship is not conducive for you. Just like you are not comfortable with everyone in the world, neither will you be comfortable with every therapist. Persist until you find someone who is a good fit for you. If you do not feel the person you talked with will be acceptable for you, simply say, "I do not believe we are a good fit. Thank you for your time."

A well-working relationship with your therapist is a G-dsend. A bad relationship is a waste of your time, energy, and money. There are many choices. Make sure your prospective therapist has a communication style that is compatible with you and that you are comfortable with the person.

Good communication and comfortableness with a therapist does not mean they will not challenge you about your thought processes or decision-making. Asking hard questions is part of their job. Get used to being uncomfortable occasionally, or sometimes being told you are wrong. Your therapist is your guide, not your buddy.

If you cannot afford a therapist, call a local or state social services agency. Tell them you have autism and that you do not have the money to pay for a therapist. Ask if there is someone you can see for free or on a sliding scale, meaning that payment is determined by how much money you are able to pay.

Be smart. Walk with a guide in the forest if you need one. It is natural and normal to get help. If you feel the world is too much, a good therapist can help rescue you from your pain, confusion, and depression.

Chapter 22

It's OK to Be Different (Follow Your Own Path)

It's OK to be different – it really is.

When I was a child, my mother used to ask, "If everyone else jumps off a bridge, will you do it too?" Thoughtless people follow the crowd, afraid to think for themselves. Brave, courageous souls follow their own hearts and brains, and walk their own paths in life.

It is easy to follow the faceless crowd because you want to fit in; it takes boldness to discover your own unique trail.

When you walk your own path, you will discover your own truths and what is truly important to you. When you allow yourself to be distinctive, you will evolve into who you are meant to be. By choosing to follow your own path, you will shine and be able to share your gifts with the world.

Here are a few examples of ways you can share your personal light with the world:

1. While volunteering in a hospital, sit down and talk to a lonely patient.
2. Volunteer at a school or daycare center and help teach the children to read.
3. Take food to a sick neighbor.

There are endless possibilities and opportunities to share your gifts with others.

You did not come to Earth to be selfish and shut off from everyone.

You were born to share and allow your light to brighten the world.

What happens if you choose to stay closed up in your room or house? Your gift will wither away like a flower trying to survive the hot desert sun.

The choice is yours, so what will it be? Will you choose to follow the crowd, or be brave, become your own individual person, and shine your personal light out into the world?

Break out of your box and follow your own unique path.

Chapter 23

Don't Be a Sucker

Autistics are naive. It's difficult to admit, but it's true. We are honest to a fault and surprised when the rest of the world is not. Because we are honest when we deal with others, we expect them to be fair with us, too. This is **not** how the neurotypical world works. Because we are always honest, they sometimes think we are stupid. And sometimes we are.

Let me give you an example from my own life. A woman I met who worked at a grocery store became friendly with me very quickly. After a short while, she asked to borrow $200 because she was short on her rent payment. She promised to pay me back in three or four days. I trusted her. She offered no collateral I could keep if she did not repay the loan. Because I barely knew her, it was not a good idea to loan her money. Fortunately, she paid me back.

We hadn't talked for a long time when this same woman reappeared in my life. We hung out numerous times together. One day, she called me on the phone and said she needed to borrow a lot of money. She wouldn't tell me how much until I saw her. When I arrived at her apartment later that day, she shocked me with the numbers. She had racked up more than $4,000 on one credit card. A second credit card was charged up to $5,500 with expensive furniture that, for a period of time, would be interest-free for her. In two months, she would begin paying a very high amount of interest for her furniture. And, if I was really generous (and stupid), I could help pay off her truck. That would be an additional $20,000. Even though she couldn't afford to pay interest on her credit cards, she promised to pay me a lot of interest and, of course, pay me back quickly. Wisely, I did not take her up on her $29,500 petition for help. I thought about it, which was bad enough. I am not a bank. She very easily could have left me high and dry and feeling very, very stupid.

This woman is nice and works very hard. She may not have intended to take advantage of me, but she very easily could have. She might have had every intention of paying me back, but I was smart enough to realize that life could have gotten in her way and prevented her from doing so.

Before she asked me to borrow money, that same woman suggested that I shave all my body hair so I could attract a woman. EVERY BIT of body hair. I am happy I didn't follow her advice. My concept of self would have been shattered.

I feel embarrassed to admit that someone I trusted tried to take advantage of me. That experience taught me to be very careful and hope that people I do not know well will keep their word.

A number of neurotypicals see us as suckers, perhaps because we try so hard to be friends. There seem to be "victim" stickers on our foreheads. I go to ridiculous lengths to help others. In *Chapter 11: How to Develop Friendships*, I mentioned a woman who wanted to purchase a new car. She didn't need money from me; she wanted me to research everything for her: how much she should be paying, where to find the exterior/interior she wanted, and to generally consult with her about all the other details. After a while, she complained that I was "pushing" her too much. I, on the other hand, felt she was pressuring me for answers every day.

Finally, I decided to give full control of the process back to her. I would stay out of the picture until she asked for help with a specific problem. Only a husband or her father would have helped her as much as I did. I didn't even have a chance of being in a relationship with her; she made that clear before she asked for my help. So why was I doing all that work? To gain her friendship and trust. I thought that if I helped her purchase a car, she would change her mind about being in a relationship with me. She did not.

Not understanding subtext, the real meaning behind words, can also contribute to communication problems. When the woman I helped buy the car was texting me dozens of times a day, she would put smiley faces and exclamation points at the end of her sentences. I interpreted those symbols to indicate that she was happy. She wasn't. I couldn't tell she was unhappy until we talked on the phone when I could hear the exasperation in her voice. An autistic would just tell you they weren't happy. Neurotypicals expect you to know that they are dissatisfied.

What can we do to prevent people from taking advantage of us? Stop going to the ends of the earth for a friend, or someone you are hoping will be your friend, if you only do what you think (or what they tell you) they want. **Have a boundary of self-respect.** Someone who is willing to be your friend will spend time with you because they like being around you. You don't have to give them all your time and energy. Time is of a limited supply. Share yours with those who are true friends. Don't give your time away freely for nothing in return.

Autistics also share way too much information with people they barely know. This can make the other person feel uncomfortable. I know, we are only trying to be honest and not hide anything. But when we reveal too much too soon, we do not know if we can trust the other person to keep our secrets. On top of that, they may feel awkward because they may feel obligated to share more than they want to before a sense of trust has developed between you and them. Trust takes time to build; it is not immediate.

Another problem we have is that we are always exact, and expect others to do what they say, or what we think they should do. Don't look at the world as either black or white. Most of it is in the gray middle. When you are a passenger in a car, don't get upset when the driver is going five miles per hour above the speed limit. It's OK. If a family member says they will call you at 10 a.m. don't give them a difficult time because they *finally* call you at 10:20 a.m. Only autistics are this exact. We need to learn that most of the world works in the gray area.

When something is important to you, share it with the other person. For example, if you have a job interview on the phone at 3:30 p.m., tell the family member who promised to call you at 3 p.m. about the scheduled interview. If they call you during the job interview, it is OK to be unhappy because you informed the family member about your impending important phone call 30 minutes past the time they were supposed to call you. They need to be considerate.

Step out of the sucker box.

Let me share with you the things a good friend does for another friend:

- Listens
- Shares their thoughts
- Helps in appropriate ways (e.g., if your acquaintance is moving, help them move boxes, not plan the move)
- Does fun things together

Trust and time build friendships, not going to extremes like doing all the research necessary to buy a car early on in a friendship or allowing someone you barely know to borrow money. **You are worthy of having a friend for the simple reason that you are a good friend.**

Stand up for yourself. Do not allow others to take advantage, as you will be very upset if that occurs. Take your time becoming friends. Learn who they are and avoid sharing personal information too early in the relationship. Maybe you will become best friends, maybe casual friends. Only time will tell.

Chapter 24

Be Wise

Your parents, teachers, and other important people in your life are not always correct. Yes, it is important to listen to them. They often will guide you in the right direction. But, not always.

In 2003, I drove to Phoenix from St. Louis to meet a woman with whom I had been corresponding with all summer, and to see my father. To my shock, he had lost 50 pounds in one month because he had diarrhea and barely ate. He was in very poor health.

I talked him into seeing his doctor, which we did a few days later. His physician examined him and took bloodwork. One or two days after the appointment, the doctor's office called both of us to inform us that the doctor wanted to see my father a few days later, on Friday afternoon. When I saw my father in his apartment, he was banging his closed fist on the kitchen table and growled that he would not go back for a second appointment.

That upset me. What occurred the next day was much worse. When I was back in my father's apartment, he told me he had attempted to kill himself by putting a plastic bag over his head, but he had failed because he'd been too scared about being unable to breathe. He wanted my help with keeping the bag over his head so he could succeed with the suicide.

That was terrifying. Rather than telling my father I didn't want him to die, I told him that if I did what he wanted me to do I would wind up in prison. Fortunately, he immediately changed his mind and decided not to die.

After I spoke with him the next day, he chose to see his doctor for a second appointment. Another blood test was taken. This time, the results were immediately available. My father was told he needed to go to the hospital very quickly or he would be dead in one or two days.

My father recovered a few weeks later. He lived for another three years and five months. He died because he had cancer throughout his body, including his brain. I was with him in a hospice home for the last 10 hours before he died. His last words were, "I love you."

I was fortunate that I did not kill my father, even though he said he wanted me to, and that we were able to see his doctor for a second appointment. Sometimes in life, we must follow our gut instincts. In this case, I would have been haunted nearly every minute of my life if I had helped my father die. I also would have been unable to help others because I would have been in prison for a very long time. My entire world would have changed in a very bad way.

Chapter 25

Happiness

How does one create a happy heart? By focusing on our dreams, or goals, in life.

In *Chapter 3: Dreams and Aspirations*, I wrote, "Without dreams, we live our lives aimlessly." We are all on this Earth to work hard and do the best we can. In the same chapter, I explained how to reach our dreams: through encouragement, hope, and constructing a plan.

Our dreams, or goals, might be easy or difficult to attain. It doesn't matter how easy or hard they are to achieve. What matters is the effort we put into reaching our dreams. Sometimes we can complete our goals; other times we cannot.

My dream has always been to help others. This is why I worked as a reporter for weekly and daily newspapers and volunteered for numerous organizations beginning in high school. While working in a small town in Missouri, I took a picture of a high school student who was donating blood to the Red Cross. Before his process began, a group of other students was harassing him. I hope the picture I took of him that was published in the newspaper made him feel better.

In high school, I was the head volunteer of a small group of students who served older adults dinner once a month in our religious building. While they were eating, I also played piano for them. Helping others in small or large ways is important to me.

In *Chapter 15: Eliminate Sadness*, I wrote, "Sadness is common for those with autism because we are alone in life, even when we do not want to be." Working on reaching our dreams will help eliminate our sadness.

Another way to build happiness is by being close to others, be they family or friends. Helping another person, including sharing thoughts and feelings, can bring you closer to them. You might be surprised to learn how sharing your feelings, or listening to a family member or friend, could change their life in a positive manner.

Step out of your box and move toward a happy heart.

Chapter 26

Concluding Thoughts

Those of us on the autism spectrum want the same things that neurotypicals desire: fulfillment, love, feeling we make a difference in the world, productive work, and friends. We have a much more difficult time reaching our dreams because of our lower level of communication skills compared to those who do not have autism.

In this book, I have tried to explain the difficulties those with autism have when it comes to dealing with the outside world and how to hurdle over those challenges. Reaching our goals requires us to work together with everyone – autistics and neurotypicals. I also hope this book has helped neurotypicals understand our challenges so they will be willing to meet us halfway or more, particularly if we cannot move very close to the center.

This does not mean that those with autism can sit back and let others do all the changing and compromising while we stay in our comfort zone. We must be a part of the solution by communicating and making an effort to reach as close to the center as we can. We may not be able to move far, but we must do the best we can.

It is OK to be different from the crowd, to do your own thing and see the world your way. We are all unique because we are individuals. But because we are a part of society, sometimes we have to take steps we would rather not take.

Neurotypicals must realize that at times autistics cannot move toward what they need, e.g., picking up on social cues. It can take decades, like it did for me, to uncover what I was missing because those with autism don't naturally understand subtext, body language, and other social cues. For some autistic people, particular social skills may never develop. Everyone has their own set of limitations.

Sometimes I wish neurotypicals would accept me for who I am without thinking I am "eccentric." Yes, I am different from those not on the spectrum. Neurotypicals are very dissimilar from me, but I accept them for who they are and try to work with them from across the aisle, as they say in politics.

Those on the autism spectrum are responsible for their lives. Try your best in everything you do, be it in school, at work, making friends, or being in a relationship. Do not become frustrated if you do not reach your every goal; no one does. But never give up making the attempt. You can only grow if you make an effort to reach your goals.

Move out of your box and reach for the stars. You will go far beyond your most imaginative dreams.

Endnotes

1   Adults with Asperger Syndrome, autism-help.org

2   https://www.cdc.gov/ncbddd/autism/features/adults-living-with-autism-spectrum-disorder.html

3   *American Psychiatric Association: Diagnostic and Statistical Manual of Mental Disorders*, Fifth Edition. Arlington, VA, American Psychiatric Association, 2013.

4   Ibid.

5   Adults with Asperger Syndrome, autism-help.org

6   *American Psychiatric Association: Diagnostic and Statistical Manual of Mental Disorders*, Fifth Edition. Arlington, VA, American Psychiatric Association, 2013.

7   Austin, Grace, "Is It Time for Asperger's in the Workplace?" *Diversity Journal*, Nov. 29, 2012 diversityjournal.com

8   Roux, Anne M., Shattuck, Paul T., Rast, Jessica E., Rava, Julianna A., and Anderson, Kristy, A. *National Autism Indicators Report: Transition into Young Adulthood*. Philadelphia, PA: Life Course Outcomes Research Program, A.J. Drexel Autism Institute, Drexel University, 2015, p. 35.

9   Ibid, p. 14.

10   Ibid, p. 32.

11   Ibid, p. 65.

12   Ibid.

13   https://www.cdc.gov/ncbddd/autism/data.html

14 Maenner MJ, Warren Z, Williams AR, et al. Prevalence and Characteristics of Autism Spectrum Disorder Among Children Aged 8 Years-Autism and Developmental Disabilities Monitoring Network, 11 sites, United States, 2020. MMWR Surveill Summ 2023; 72 (No. SS-2): 1-14. DOI: http://dx.doi.org/10.15585/mmwr.ss7202a1

15 Ibid.

16 Ibid.

17 https://web.archive.org/web/20160510205435/https://cdc.gov/ncbddd/autism/research.html

18 Ibid.

19 Maenner MJ, Warren Z, Williams AR, et al. Prevalence and Characteristics of Autism Spectrum Disorder Among Children Aged 8 Years-Autism and Developmental Disabilities Monitoring Network, 11 sites, United States, 2020. MMWR Surveill Summ 2023; 72 (No. SS-2): 1-14. DOI: http://dx.doi.org/10.15585/mmwr.ss7202a1

20 https://www.cdc.gov/ncbddd/autism/addm-network-funding.html

21 https://www.cdc.gov/ncbddd/autism/features/adults-living-with-autism-spectrum-disorder.html

22 Ibid.

23 Roux, Anne M., Shattuck, Paul T., Rast, Jessica E., Rava, Julianna A., and Anderson, Kristy, A. *National Autism Indicators Report: Transition into Young Adulthood*. Philadelphia, PA: Life Course Outcomes Research Program, A.J. Drexel Autism Institute, Drexel University, 2015, p. 35.

24 *American Psychiatric Association: Diagnostic and Statistical Manual of Mental Disorders*, Fifth Edition. Arlington, VA, American Psychiatric Association, 2013.

25 "Sweeping study underscores autism's overlap with obsessions," by Ann Griswold, Dec. 3, 2015, spectrumnews.org

26 *American Psychiatric Association: Diagnostic and Statistical Manual of Mental Disorders*, Fifth Edition. Arlington, VA, American Psychiatric Association, 2013.

27 Cassidy, S., et. al. Suicidal ideation and suicide plans or attempts in adults with Asperger's Syndrome attending a specialist diagnostic clinic: a clinical cohort study. *The Lancet Psychiatry,* June 24, 2014.

28 Ibid.

www.ingramcontent.com/pod-product-compliance
Lightning Source LLC
Chambersburg PA
CBHW052032030426
42337CB00027B/4971